Synopsis On Spinal Injuries

Gourishankar Patnaik
MBBS,MS(Orth)FAOI(USA)MA(PubAdmn,Socio,Eco)PhD
Kumar Anshuman
MBBS,DNB(Ortho)
Department of Orthopedics,Trauma and Rehabilitation
Narayan Medical College Jamuhar, Bihar ,INDIA

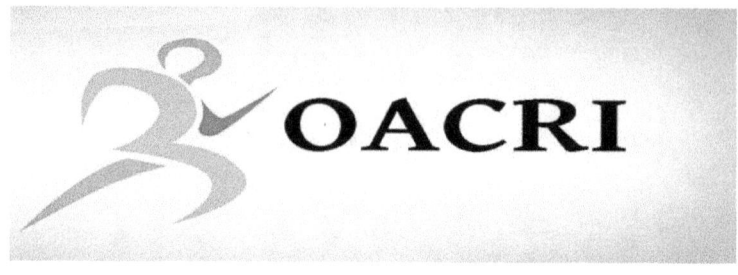

OSTEOPOROSIS AND OSTEOARTHRITIS CARE AND RESEARCH INITIATIVE

A MEDICAL COMMUNICATIOS GROUP

Published in the USA

Copyright © [2014] by [Gourishankar Patnaik]
All rights reserved.
ISBN-13: **978-1505725568**
ISBN-10: **1505725569**
BISAC: **Medical / Orthopedics**

No part of this publicationmay be reproduced, stored in a retrieval systemor transmitted, in any form or by any means, without the prior permission in writing from oacri group of publications

DEDICATED TO

Members of our family who supported us, the medical students and most importantly the numerous patients who have reposed faith in us.

Index

Chapter 1	Introduction
Chapter 2	Normal Spinal Cord
Chapter 3	Spinal Injuries-The Syndrome
Chapter 4	Physiological Changes after Injury
Chapter 5	Secondary Injures
Chapter 6	Regeneration
Chapter 7	Management of spinal Cord Injuries
Chapter 8	Newer Inventions
Chapter 9	Rehabilitation
Chapter 10	Conclusion

About Authors

Books written by Author

Preface

As the 21st century begins to bloom, advances in scientific understanding of the human body are leading to tremendous opportunities for treating even the most devastating diseases. Among the most exciting frontiers in medicine is the repair of traumatic injuries to the central nervous system (CNS), including the spinal cord. Improvements in treatment are helping many more people survive spinal cord injury, and the time survivors must spend in the hospital is half what it was 20 years ago. Yet most spinal cord injuries still cause lifelong disability, and further research is critically needed. The injury of actor Christopher Reeve in 1995 drew the world's attention to the tragedy of spinal cord injury. The incidence of spinal cord injuries peaks among people in their early 20s, with a small increase in the elderly population due to falls and degenerative diseases of the spine. Because spinal cord injuries usually occur in early adulthood, those affected often require costly supportive care for many decades. The individual costs may exceed $250,000 per year, placing an often overwhelming financial burden on these individuals and their families.

Spinal cord injuries and its aftereffect create enormous burden to the families who become victims of the aftereffects of these disastrous injuries. The consequences are social, economical, and psychological besides medical and surgical complications. Attempt has been made to portray the larger picture of these injuries and its various ramifications. It is primarily intended for the medical students and general practiotioners in understanding of these complex injuries.

Gourishankar Patnaik   Jamuhar, India

Kumar Anshuman

Chapter 1

Introduction

As the 21st century begins to bloom, advances in scientific understanding of the human body are leading to tremendous opportunities for treating even the most devastating diseases. Among the most exciting frontiers in medicine is the repair of traumatic injuries to the central nervous system (CNS), including the spinal cord. Improvements in treatment are helping many more people survive spinal cord injury, and the time survivors must spend in the hospital is half what it was 20 years ago. Yet most spinal cord injuries still cause lifelong disability, and further research is critically needed.

The injury of actor Christopher Reeve in 1995 drew the world's attention to the tragedy of spinal cord injury. Accidents and violence cause an estimated 10,000 spinal cord injuries each year, and more than 200,000 Americans live day-to-day with the disabling effects of such trauma. The incidence of spinal cord injuries peaks among people in their early 20s, with a small increase in the elderly population due to falls and degenerative diseases of the spine. Because spinal cord injuries usually occur in early adulthood, those affected often require costly supportive care for many decades. The individual costs may exceed $250,000 per year, placing an often overwhelming financial burden on these individuals and their families. For the nation, these costs add up to an estimated $10 billion per year for medical and supportive care alone. Of course, no dollar figure can describe the human costs to spinal cord injured people and their families.

Experts from the field of spinal cord injury research and leaders from other fields such as development, immunology, and stroke constantly work with the hope that those interactions among these experts might bring new interest and new ideas to spinal cord injury research and foster fruitful collaborations between investigators. Because of the remarkable progress in basic and clinical neuroscience, the time is now ripe to apply knowledge from other fields to treatment of spinal cord injury.

- Each year an estimated 11,000 Americans sustain spinal cord injuries (SCI). Nearly 250,000 people who have sustained spinal cord injuries are currently living in the United States
- The majority of people who sustain spinal cord injuries are between the ages of 16 and 30, and the average age at the time of injury is between 29.7 years and 33.4 years
- The most frequent age at which spinal cord injuries occur is 19 years. Men suffer from spinal cord injuries more frequently than women in a ratio of 4:1

- The most common causes of spinal cord injuries are motor vehicle accidents (35%-44%), violence (24%-30%), falls (19%-22%), sports related injuries of which diving accidents account for 2/3 of the injuries (7%-8%), work related and other accidents (2%-8%).

- After age 45, falls account for more spinal cord injuries than motor vehicle accidents

- While the overall incidence of spinal cord injuries is decreasing, the number of injuries that are results of violence are increasing

Four major topics for discussion:

- The current understanding and treatment of spinal cord injury
- Mechanisms of secondary damage
- Possibilities for regeneration, and
- Strategies for intervention.

In recent years scientists have gained a better understanding of how trauma injures nerve cells and why cells die. They know that secondary damage continues for hours following an initial trauma, presenting windows of opportunity to limit this damage. Other opportunities for therapeutic intervention, including rehabilitation strategies, extend well beyond this time window. Progress in understanding how the spinal cord changes after injury are pointing to new therapeutic approaches.

The ultimate hope, of course, is not just to minimize damage, but to foster recovery. A century of pessimism about the capacity for regeneration in the brain and spinal cord is now giving way to guarded optimism. Scientists recently demonstrated that nerve cells in the spinal cord can regrow under certain circumstances. Insights from animal models of spinal cord injury and from studies of nervous system development are leading to strategies that may foster regeneration. Researchers also are making outstanding progress in devising neural prostheses that can substitute for some of the functions lost after spinal cord injury. While it is unlikely that the complex problem of spinal cord injury will be solved by a single dramatic discovery, small improvements in therapy can combine to improve the quality of life for those who live with such devastating injuries.

Research in spinal cord regeneration is catching attention of clinicians and basic scientists. It would almost revolutionise the life and disease outcome of these unfortunate patients if we can work out a cost effective and practical treatment regimen for these victims who are unfortunately in the prime of their productive years. It was gratifying to learn that nerves in peripheral nervous system (PNS), which are outside the brain or spinal cord, did regrow. It is exciting to learn that the prospects of regrowth of spinal cord improves when these PNS cells are implanted in damaged spinal cord. Spinal cord injury is a global epidemic. A lot of research is going on in this field. Axonal regeneration, electric stimulation, Netrins, stem cells etc are few exciting fields in the area of research. It is ongoing research whereby the ability to grow human motor neurons in the laboratory will provide new insights into disease processes and could be used as alternative to animal models for finding therapeutic targets and testing drug.

Chapter 2

The Normal Spinal Cord

The spinal cord and the brain together make up the CNS. The spinal cord coordinates the body's movement and sensation. Unlike nerve cells, or neurons, of the peripheral nervous system (PNS), which carry signals to the limbs, torso, and other parts of the body, neurons of the CNS do not regenerate after injury.

The spinal cord includes nerve cells, or neurons, and long nerve fibers called axons. Axons in the spinal cord carry signals downward from the brain (along descending pathways) and upward toward the brain (along ascending pathways). Many axons in these pathways are covered by sheaths of an insulating substance called myelin, which gives them a whitish appearance; therefore, the region in which they lie is called "white matter." The nerve cells themselves, with their tree-like branches called dendrites that receive signals from other nerve cells, make up "gray matter." This gray matter lies in a butterfly-shaped region in the center of the spinal cord. Like the brain, the spinal cord is enclosed in three membranes (meninges): the pia mater, the innermost layer; the arachnoid, a delicate middle layer; and the dura mater, which is a tougher outer layer.

The spinal cord is organized into segments along its length. Nerves from each segment connect to specific regions of the body. The segments in the neck, or cervical region, referred to as C1 through C8, control signals to the neck, arms, and hands. Those in the thoracic or upper back region (T1 through T12) relay signals to the torso and some parts of the arms. Those in the upper lumbar or mid-back region just below the ribs (L1 through L5) control signals to the hips and legs. Finally, the sacral segments (S1 through S5) lie just below the lumbar segments in the mid-back and control signals to the groin, toes, and some parts of the legs. The effects of spinal cord injury at different segments reflect this organization.

Several types of cells carry out spinal cord functions. Large motor neurons have long axons that control skeletal muscles in the neck, torso, and limbs. Sensory neurons called dorsal root ganglion cells, whose axons form the nerves that carry information from the body into the spinal cord, are found immediately outside the spinal cord. Spinal interneurons, which lie completely within the spinal cord, help integrate sensory information and generate coordinated signals that control muscles. Glia, or supporting cells, far outnumber neurons in the brain and spinal cord and perform many essential functions.

One type of glial cell, the oligodendrocyte, creates the myelin sheaths that insulate axons and improve the speed and reliability of nerve signal transmission. Other glia enclose the spinal cord like the rim and spokes of a wheel, providing compartments for the ascending and descending nerve fiber tracts. Astrocytes, large star-shaped glial cells, regulate the composition of the fluids that surround nerve cells. Some of these cells also form scar tissue after injury. Smaller cells called microglia also become activated in response to injury and help clean up waste products.

All of these glial cells produce substances that support neuron survival and influence axon growth. However, these cells may also impede recovery following injury.

C1-C6	Neck flexors
C1-T1	Neck extensors
C3, C4, C5	Supply diaphragm (mostly C4)
C5, C6	Shoulder movement, raise arm (deltoid); flexion of elbow (biceps); **C6** externally rotates the arm (supinates)
C6, C7	Extends elbow and wrist (triceps and wrist extensors); pronates wrist
C7, T1	Flexes wrist
C7, T1	Supply small muscles of the hand
T1 -T6	Intercostals and trunk above the waist
T7-L1	Abdominal muscles
L1, L2, L3, L4	Thigh flexion
L2, L3, L4	Thigh adduction
L4, L5, S1	Thigh abduction
L5, S1, S2	Extension of leg at the hip (gluteus maximus)

L2, L3, L4	Extension of leg at the knee (quadriceps femoris)
L4, L5, S1, S2	Flexion of leg at the knee (hamstrings)
L4, L5, S1	Dorsiflexion of foot (tibialis anterior)
L4, L5, S1	Extension of toes
L5, S1, S2	Plantar flexion of foot
L5, S1, S2	Flexion of toes

The spinal cord is composed of many neurons, axons, and supporting cells .In addition, it must have many trophic factors in order to grow and function properly.

Neurons- nerve cells that provide the communication pathway through the body. There are as many as 10,000 subtypes of neurons which are specialized to receive and send information detect changes in the environment, and organize immediate and long-term responses to change. Each neuron is made up of a cell body, axons, and dendrites The nucleus is located in the cell body which, along with the dendrites and <u>neuroglial cells</u> makes up the butterfly shaped "gray matter" in the center of the spinal cord. Nerve cells of the brain and spinal cord respond to insults differently from most other cells of the body, including those in the PNS. The brain and spinal cord (i.e., the CNS) are confined within bony cavities that protect them, but also render them vulnerable to compression damage caused by swelling or forceful injury. Cells of the CNS have a very high rate of metabolism and rely upon blood glucose for energy. The "safety factor," that is the extent to which normal blood flow exceeds the minimum required for healthy functioning, is much smaller in the CNS than in other tissues. For these reasons, CNS cells are particularly vulnerable to reductions in blood flow (ischemia). Other unique features of the CNS are the "blood-brain-barrier" and the "blood-spinal-cord barrier." These barriers, formed by cells lining blood vessels in the CNS, protect nerve cells by restricting entry of potentially harmful substances and cells of the immune system. Trauma may compromise these barriers, perhaps contributing to further damage in the brain and spinal cord. The blood-spinal-cord barrier also prevents entry of some potentially therapeutic drugs. Finally, in the brain and spinal cord, the glia and the extracellular matrix (the material that surrounds cells) differ from those in peripheral nerves. Each of these differences between the PNS and CNS contributes to their different responses to injury.

Chapter 3

Spinal Injury-The syndrome

Scientists are developing therapies for neurological disorders, including spinal cord injuries (SCI), brain trauma, and neurodegenerative diseases such as ALS, Huntington's and Alzheimer's diseases

The brain, spinal cord and optic nerves comprise the central nervous system (CNS) one of the most complex and enigmatic systems in nature. The CNS is responsible for consciousness, memory, intelligence, the five senses, and controlled movement. However, these functions may be disrupted by brain damage, spinal injury or disease, causing severe disability, such as paralysis, blindness, or loss of mental capabilities. The disability is often permanent because the CNS has a very limited capacity for healing and self repair.

While there is no paralysis cure yet available to treat spinal cord injury, nor any cure for CNS trauma in general, scientists at the Weizmann Institute of Science and Proneuron have demonstrated that CNS recovery may be enhanced by applying the body's own repair system, the immune system, which is actively involved in wound-healing in other parts of the body. In the quest for a paralysis cure, Proneuron is pursuing an aggressive research and development program based on proprietary immune-modulating technology. Proneuron's lead product is ProCord, an experimental cell therapy that is being developed to treat acute spinal cord injury. Besides spinal cord injuries, additional products are being developed for other debilitating neurological indications.

The American Spinal Injury Association (ASIA) defined an international classification based on neurological responses, touch and pinprick sensations tested in each dermatome, and strength of ten key muscles on each side of the body, e.g. shoulder shrug (C4), elbow flexion (C5), wrist extension (C6), elbow extension (C7), hip flexion (L2). Traumatic spinal cord injury is classified into five categories by the American Spinal Injury Association and the

International Spinal Cord Injury Classification System:

- A indicates a "complete" spinal cord injury where no motor or sensory function is preserved in the sacral segments S4-S5.
- B indicates an "incomplete" spinal cord injury where sensory but not motor function is preserved below the neurological level and includes the sacral segments S4-S5. This is typically a transient phase and if the person recovers any motor function below the neurological level, that person essentially becomes a motor incomplete, i.e. ASIA C or D.
- C indicates an "incomplete" spinal cord injury where motor function is

preserved below the neurological level and more than half of key muscles below the neurological level have a muscle grade of less than 3, which indicates active movement with full range of motion against gravity.

- D indicates an "incomplete" spinal cord injury where motor function is preserved below the neurological level and at least half of the key muscles below the neurological level have a muscle grade of 3 or more.
- E indicates "normal" where motor and sensory scores are normal. Note that it is possible to have spinal cord injury and neurological deficits with completely normal motor and sensory scores.

In addition, there are several clinical syndromes associated with incomplete spinal cord injuries.

- The Central cord syndrome is associated with greater loss of upper limb function compared to lower limbs.
- The Brown-Séquard syndrome results from injury to one side with the spinal cord, causing weakness and loss of proprioception on the side of the injury and loss of pain and thermal sensation of the other side.
- The Anterior cord syndrome results from injury to the anterior part of the spinal cord, causing weakness and loss of pain and thermal sensations below the injury site but preservation of

proprioception that is usually carried in the posterior part of the spinal cord.
- Tabes Dorsalis results from injury to the posterior part of the spinal cord, usually from infection diseases such as syphilis, causing loss of touch and proprioceptive sensation.
- Conus medullaris syndrome results from injury to the tip of the spinal cord, located at L1 vertebra.
- Cauda equina syndrome is, strictly speaking, not really spinal cord injury but injury to the spinal roots below the L1 vertebra.

Facts and Figures

One can have spine injury without spinal cord injury. Many people suffer transient loss of function ("stingers") in sports accidents or pain in "whiplash" of the neck without neurological loss and relatively few of these suffer spinal cord injury sufficient to warrant hospitalization. In the United States, the incidence of spinal cord injury has been estimated to be about 40 cases (per 1 million people) per year or 12,000 cases per year. In China, the incidence of spinal cord injury is approximately 60,000 per year.

The prevalence of spinal cord injury is not well known in many large countries. In some countries, such as Sweden and Iceland, registries are available. According to new data collected by the Christopher and Dana Reeve Foundation, in the US, there are currently 1.3 million individuals living with spinal cord injuries- a number five times that previously estimated in 2007. 61% of spinal cord injuries occur in males, and 39% in females. The average age for spinal cord injuries is 48 years old. There are many causes leading to spinal cord injuries. These include motor vehicle accidents (24%), work-related accidents (28%), and sporting /recreation accidents (16%), and falls (9%)

The effects of a spinal cord injury may vary depending on the type, level, and severity of injury, but can be classified into two general categories:

- In a *complete injury*, function below the "neurological" level is lost. Absence of motor and sensory function below a specific spinal level is considered a "complete injury". Recent evidence suggests that less than 5% of people with "complete" spinal cord injuries recover locomotion.

- In an *incomplete injury*, some sensation and/or movement below the level of the injury is retained. The lowest spinal segment in humans is located at vertebral levels S4-5, corresponding to the anal sphincter and peri-anal sensation. The ability to contract the anal sphincter voluntarily or to feel peri-anal pinprick or touch, the injury is considered to be "incomplete". Recent evidence suggests that over 95% of people with "incomplete" spinal cord injuries recover some locomotor function.

In addition to loss of sensation and motor function below the level of injury, individuals with spinal cord injuries will also often experience other complications:

- Bowel and bladder function is regulated by the sacral region of the spine. In that regard, it is very common to experience dysfunction of the bowel and bladder, including infections of the bladder and anal incontinence, after traumatic injury.
- Sexual function is also associated with the sacral spinal segments, and is often affected after injury. During a psychogenic sexual experience, signals

from the brain are sent to spinal levels T10-L2 and in case of men, are then relayed to the penis where they trigger an erection. A reflex erection, on the other hand, occurs as a result of direct physical contact to the penis or other erotic areas such as the ears, nipples or neck. A reflex erection is involuntary and can occur without sexually stimulating thoughts. The nerves that control a man's ability to have a reflex erection are located in the sacral nerves (S2-S4) of the spinal cord and could be affected after a spinal cord injury.[5]

- Injuries at the C-1/C-2 levels will often result in loss of breathing,

necessitating mechanical ventilators or phrenic nerve pacing.
- Inability or reduced ability to regulate heart rate, blood pressure, sweating and hence body temperature.
- Spasticity (increased reflexes and stiffness of the limbs).
- Neuropathic pain.
- Autonomic dysreflexia or abnormal increases in blood pressure, sweating, and other autonomic responses to pain or sensory disturbances.
- Atrophy of muscle.
- Superior Mesenteric Artery Syndrome.
- Osteoporosis (loss of calcium) and bone degeneration.
- Gallbladder and renal stones.

The Location of the Injury

Determining the exact level of injury is critical in making accurate predictions about the specific parts of the body that may be affected by paralysis and loss of function.

The symptoms observed after a spinal cord injury differ by location (refer to the spinal cord map on the right to determine location). Notably, while the prognosis of complete injuries are generally predictable, the symptoms of incomplete injuries span a variable range. Accordingly, it is difficult to make an accurate prognosis for these types of injuries.

Cervical injuries

Cervical (neck) injuries usually result in full or partial tetraplegia (Quadriplegia). However, depending on the specific location and severity of trauma, limited function may be retained.

- **C3 vertebrae and above** : Typically results in loss of diaphragm function, necessitating the use of a ventilator for breathing.
- **C4 :** Results in significant loss of function at the biceps and shoulders.
- **C5** : Results in potential loss of function at the shoulders and biceps, and complete loss of function at the wrists and hands.

- ***C6**: Results in limited wrist control, and* complete loss of hand function.
- **C7 and T1**: Results in lack of dexterity in the hands and fingers, but allows for limited use of arms. C7 is generally the threshold level for retaining functional independence.

Thoracic injuries

Injuries at or below the thoracic spinal levels result in paraplegia. Function of the hands, arms, neck, and breathing is usually not affected.

- **T1 to T8**: Results in the inability to control the abdominal muscles. Accordingly, trunk stability is affected. The lower the level of injury, the less severe the effects.

- **T9 to T12**: Results in partial loss of trunk and abdominal muscle control.

Lumbar and Sacral injuries

The effects of injuries to the lumbar or sacral regions of the spinal cord are decreased control of the legs and hips, urinary system, and anus.

Central Cord and Other Syndromes

Central cord syndrome is a form of incomplete spinal cord injury characterized by impairment in the arms and hands and, to a lesser extent, in the legs. This is also referred to as inverse paraplegia, because the hands and arms are paralyzed while the legs and lower extremities work correctly.

Most often the damage is to the cervical or upper thoracic regions of the spinal cord, and characterized by weakness in the arms with relative sparing of the legs with variable sensory loss.

This condition is associated with ischemia, hemorrhage, or necrosis involving the central portions of the spinal cord (the large nerve fibers that carry information directly from the cerebral cortex). Corticospinal fibers destined for the legs are spared due to their more external location in the spinal cord.

This clinical pattern may emerge during recovery from spinal shock due to prolonged swelling around or near the vertebrae, causing pressures on the cord. The symptoms may be transient or permanent.

Anterior cord syndrome (picture 2) is also an incomplete spinal cord injury. Below the injury, motor function, pain sensation, and temperature sensation is lost; touch, proprioception (sense of position in space), and vibration sense remain intact. Posterior cord syndrome (not pictured) can also occur, but is very rare. Brown-Séquard syndrome (picture 3) usually occurs when the spinal cord is hemisectioned or injured on the lateral side. On the ipsilateral side of the injury (same side), there is a loss of motor function, proprioception, vibration, and light touch. Contralaterally (opposite side of injury), there is a loss of pain, temperature, and deep touch sensations

Treatment

Treatment options for acute, traumatic non-penetrating spinal cord injuries include the administration of a high dose of an anti-inflammatory agent, methylprednisolone, within 8 hours of injury. This recommendation is primarily based on the National Acute Spinal Cord Injury Studies (NASCIS) I and II. However, in a third study, methylprednisolone failed to demonstrate an effect in comparison to placebo. Additionally, due to increased risk of infections, the use of this anti-inflammatory drug after spinal cord injuries is no longer recommended [6][7]. Presently, administration of cold saline acutely after injury is gaining popularity, but there is a paucity of empirical evidence for the beneficial effects of therapeutic hypothermia.

Scientists are investigating many promising avenues for treatment of spinal cord injury. Numerous articles in the medical literature describe research, mostly in animal models, aimed at reducing the paralyzing effects of injury and promoting regrowth of functional nerve fibers. Despite the devastating effects of the condition, commercial funding for research investigating a cure after spinal cord injury is limited, partially due to the small size of the population of potential beneficiaries. Despite this limitation, a number of experimental treatments have reached controlled human trials. In addition, therapeutic strategies involving neuronal protection and regeneration are also being investigated in other neurodegenerative diseases such as Alzheimer's Disease, Parkinson's Disease, Amyotrophic Lateral Sclerosis and Multiple sclerosis. There are many similarities between these conditions of the CNS and spinal cord injuries, thus increasing the potential for discovery of a treatment after spinal cord injuries.

Advances in identification of an effective therapeutic target after spinal cord injury have been newsworthy, and considerable media attention is often drawn towards new developments in this area. However, aside from methylprednisolone, none of these developments have reached even limited use in the clinical care of human spinal cord injury in the U.S. Around the world, proprietary centers offering stem cell transplants and treatment with neuroregenerative substances are fueled by glowing testimonial reports of neurological improvement. It is also evident that when stem cells when injected in the area of damage in the spinal cord, they secrete neurotrophic factors and these neurotrophic factors help neurons and vessels grow to thus helping repair the damage. Independent validation of the results of these treatments is lacking.

Chapter 4

Anatomical and Functional Changes after Injury

Overview:

The types of disability associated with spinal cord injury vary greatly depending on the severity of the injury, the segment of the spinal cord at which the injury occurs, and which nerve fibers are damaged. In spinal cord injury, the destruction of nerve fibers that carry motor signals from the brain to the torso and limbs leads to muscle paralysis. Destruction of sensory nerve fibers can lead to loss of sensations such as touch, pressure, and temperature; it sometimes also causes pain. Other serious consequences can include exaggerated reflexes; loss of bladder and bowel control; sexual dysfunction; lost or decreased breathing capacity; impaired cough reflexes; and spasticity (abnormally strong muscle contractions). Most people with spinal cord injury regain some functions between a week and six months after injury, but the likelihood of spontaneous recovery diminishes after six months. Rehabilitation strategies can minimize the long-term disability.

Spinal cord injuries can lead to many secondary complications, including pressure sores, increased susceptibility to respiratory diseases, and autonomic dysreflexia. Autonomic dysreflexia is a potentially life-threatening increase in blood pressure, sweating, and other autonomic reflexes in reaction to bowel impaction or some other stimulus. Careful medical management and skilled supportive care is necessary to prevent these complications.

Researchers studying spinal cords obtained from autopsy have identified several different types of spinal cord injuries. The most common types of spinal cord injuries found in one large study were contusions (bruising of the spinal cord) and compression injuries (caused by pressure on the spinal cord). Other types of injury included lacerations, caused by a bullet or other object, and central cord syndrome.

Secondary Damage

Damage to the spinal cord does not stop with the initial injury, but continues in the hours following trauma. Paradoxically, this delayed, secondary damage is not all bad news because secondary injury processes present windows of time in which treatment may reduce the extent of disability. The effects of methylprednisolone demonstrate that such treatment is possible and present a model for the development of other treatments.

Two major themes about secondary damage recurred throughout the workshop. The first theme reflects increasing recognition that similar cellular processes contribute to damage in many different neurological disorders. The second theme mirrors one of the most active areas in all of biology -- how cells die. Cells, including those in the spinal cord, die in two general ways. Necrosis is a relatively uncontrolled process in which cells swell and break open, leaking substances that can be toxic to their neighbors. However, in apoptosis, or programmed cell death, cells activate a "cell suicide" program, an ordered sequence of events that leads to cell death with relatively little damage to surrounding cells. The relationship between apoptosis and necrosis, the role that each plays in spinal cord injury, the signals that regulate cell death, and the potential to halt death programs are now being explored to find ways of minimizing secondary damage following spinal cord injury.

In contusion injuries, a cavity, or hole, often forms in the center of the spinal cord. Myelinated axons typically survive in a ring along the inside edge of the cord. Some axons may survive in the center cavity, but they usually lose their myelin covering. This demyelination greatly slows the speed of nerve transmission. Slowing of nerve impulses can be measured by a diagnostic technique called transcranial magnetic stimulation (TMS).

Another example of a spinal cord injury is central cord syndrome, which affects the cervical (neck) region of the cord and results from focused damage to a group of nerve fibers called the corticospinal tract. The corticospinal tract controls movement by carrying signals between the brain and the spinal cord. Patients with central cord syndrome typically have relatively mild impairment, and they often spontaneously recover many of their abilities. Patients usually recover substantially by 6 weeks after injury, despite continued loss of axons and myelin. Delays in motor responses persist, but permanent impairment is usually confined to the hands.

Complete severing of the spinal cord is rare in humans, but even axons that survive the initial injury often lose their ability to function. Secondary damage, which continues for hours, can cause loss of myelin, degeneration of axons, and nerve cell death. Patients with their spinal cords completely severed often show abnormal reflexes that emerge more than 8 months after injury. These reflexes, such as twitching of muscles in the arm and hand in response to sensory stimulation of the legs and feet, may result from "sprouting" of new branches from sensory fibers just below the lesion. They may also result from activation of nerve pathways that are normally suppressed. Other abnormal responses, such as sweating in response to movement of a hair, may be due to sprouting of nerves in the autonomic nervous system. The autonomic nervous system is the part of the PNS that controls involuntary body functions such as sweating and heart rate. Since even a small number of nerve fibers can support significant nervous system function, measures that reduce damage could allow much greater function than would otherwise be expected. Devising interventions that will achieve this goal is one of the major challenges in spinal cord injury research today. Clinical Management

Medical care of spinal cord injury has advanced greatly in the last 50 years. During World War II, injury to the spinal cord was usually fatal. While postwar advances in emergency care and rehabilitation allowed many patients to survive, methods for reducing the extent of injury were virtually unknown. Although techniques to reduce secondary damage, such as cord irrigation and cooling, were first tried 20 to 30 years ago, the principles underlying effective use of these strategies were not well understood. Significant advances in recent years, including an effective drug therapy for acute spinal cord injury (methylprednisolone) and better imaging techniques for diagnosing spinal damage, have improved the recovery of patients with spinal cord injuries.

Current care of acute spinal cord injury involves three primary considerations. First, physicians must diagnose and relieve cord compression, gross misalignments of the spine, and other structural problems. Second, they must minimize cellular-level damage if at all possible. Finally, they must stabilize the vertebrae to prevent further injury.

The care and treatment of persons with a suspected spinal cord injury begins with emergency medical services personnel, who must evaluate and immobilize the patient. Any movement of the person, or even resuscitation efforts, could cause further injury. Even with much-improved emergency medical care, many people with spinal cord injury still die before reaching the hospital.

Methylprednisolone, a steroid, has become standard treatment for acute spinal cord injury since 1990, when a large-scale clinical trial showed significantly better recovery in patients who began treatment with this drug within 8 hours of their injury. Methylprednisolone reduces the damage to cellular membranes that contributes to neuronal death after injury. It also reduces inflammation near the injury and suppresses the activation of immune cells that appear to contribute to neuronal damage. Preventing this damage helps spare some nerve fibers that would otherwise be lost, improving the patient's recovery.

A controversial topic in the acute care of spinal cord injury is whether surgery to reduce pressure on the spinal cord and stabilize it is better than traction alone. A study in the 1970s showed that, in some cases, surgical intervention actually worsened the patient's condition. This finding prompted many physicians to become more conservative about using these techniques, although advances in care since that time have reduced the risk of complications due to surgery. While there is no proof that surgeons must operate to decompress the spinal cord within the 8-hour time window established for methylprednisolone, many believe it may help and try to do it then. Early surgery also allows earlier movement and earlier physical therapy, which are important for preventing complications and regaining as much function as possible. Use of imaging methods such as computed tomography (CT) scans to visualize fractures and magnetic resonance imaging (MRI) to image contusions, disc herniation, and other damage can help define the appropriate treatment for a particular patient. Several types of metal plates, screws, and other devices also are now available for surgically stabilizing the spine.

Once a patient's condition is stabilized, care and treatment focus on supportive care and rehabilitation strategies. Attention to supportive care can prevent many complications. For example, periodically changing the patient's position can prevent pressure sores and respiratory complications. Rehabilitation, which focuses on the patient's physical and emotional recovery, is also very important. Almost all patients with spinal cord injuries can now achieve a partial return of function with proper physical therapy that maintains flexibility and function of the muscles and joints. Physical therapy can also help reduce the risk of blood clots and boost the patient's morale, while counseling can help a person adjust emotionally to the injury and its consequences.

Conclusion

Recent years have seen many advances in understanding and treating spinal cord injury. These include the development of CT and MRI scans to visualize injuries and the use of methylprednisolone to reduce damage. However, many facets of what happens when the spinal cord is injured are still unknown. An exact description of the structural and tissue changes that occur in spinal cord injury is necessary for planning effective interventions. Studies aimed at better describing what happens following spinal cord injury may lead to improved treatments.

Chapter 5

SECONDARY INJURIES

Secondary Damage

Damage to the spinal cord does not stop with the initial injury, but continues in the hours following trauma. Paradoxically, this delayed, secondary damage is not all bad news because secondary injury processes present windows of time in which treatment may reduce the extent of disability. The effects of methylprednisolone demonstrate that such treatment is possible and present a model for the development of other treatments.

Two major themes about secondary damage recurred throughout the workshop. The first theme reflects increasing recognition that similar cellular processes contribute to damage in many different neurological disorders. The second theme mirrors one of the most active areas in all of biology --

how cells die. Cells, including those in the spinal cord, die in two general ways. Necrosis is a relatively uncontrolled process in which cells swell and break open, leaking substances that can be toxic to their neighbors. However, in apoptosis, or programmed cell death, cells activate a "cell suicide" program, an ordered sequence of events that leads to cell death with relatively little damage to surrounding cells. The relationship between apoptosis and necrosis, the role that each plays in spinal cord injury, the signals that regulate cell death, and the potential to halt death programs are now being explored to find ways of minimizing secondary damage following spinal cord injury.

Immune System Reactions

There is no single point at which to begin describing the intricately intertwined cellular and molecular events that follow spinal cord injury. However, the immune reaction is a good place to start because of its importance. Most types of immune cells enter the CNS only rarely unless it has been damaged by trauma or disease. It is not always clear to what extent immune reactions help or harm prospects for recovery, although immune reactions do appear to cause some secondary damage.

The last decade has brought extraordinary advances in understanding the immune system and its interactions with the nervous system. Using newly developed markers, scientists can identify subsets of immune cells with different functions and can monitor these cells in the nervous system. They are also beginning to understand the chemical language immune cells use to communicate. Cytokines, for example, are a diverse group of diffusible messenger molecules that control many aspects of immune cell function and also enable immune cells to influence other cells such as neurons. Cell adhesion molecules on the surfaces of cells control the traffic of immune cells into the brain and spinal cord and have other wide-ranging influences. Epithelial cells of blood vessels and various types of immune cells normally display certain cell adhesion molecules on their surface. These adhesion molecules change when blood vessel and immune cells encounter foreign molecules, sense damaged tissue in the vicinity, or detect cytokines. Advances in understanding the immune system are now being applied to learn how immune cells influence recovery from spinal cord injury.

Microglial cells, which are normally found in the CNS, have some immune functions and become activated in response to damage. Following trauma, other types immune cells react to signals from damaged tissue and changes in endothelial cells by entering the CNS. Neutrophils are the first type of immune cells to enter the CNS from the rest of the body. These cells enter the spinal cord within about 12 hours of injury and are present for about a day. About 3 days after the injury, T-cells enter the CNS. T cells have many functions in the body, including killing infected cells and regulating many aspects of the immune response; however, their function in spinal cord injury is totally unknown. The key types of immune cells in spinal cord injury appear to be macrophages and monocytes, which enter the CNS after the T-cells. These cells scavenge cellular debris. One type of macrophage, the perivascular cell, may also mediate damage to the endothelial cells that line blood vessels. It is not clear which signals control the entry of immune cells into the CNS, but changes in cell adhesion molecules most likely play an important role.

What immune cells do once they enter the damaged spinal cord is poorly understood. Some cells engulf and eliminate debris as they do during inflammation in other parts of the body.

Macrophages, monocytes, and microglial cells release a host of powerful regulatory substances that may help or hinder recovery from injury. Potentially beneficial substances released by these cells include the cytokines TGF-beta and GM-CSF (transforming growth factor-beta and granulocyte-macrophage colony-stimulating factor) and several other growth factors. Apparently detrimental products include cytokines such as TNF-alpha and IL-1-beta (tumor necrosis factor-alpha and interleukin-1-beta) and chemicals such as superoxides and nitric oxide that may contribute to oxidative damage. Again, it is unclear what is helpful and harmful about many of these powerful substances in the context of the injured spinal cord.

Several workshop participants emphasized how important it is to learn about the role of the immune response in spinal cord injury. Understanding the possible links between the immune system and oxidative damage, apoptosis of nerve cells, and demyelination is an important area for research. Other critical areas for study include the signals controlling the traffic of immune cells into the spinal cord following injury and the time course and subsets of immune cells involved. Progress in understanding the immune system now makes answering these questions technically possible.

Oxidative Damage

After a spinal cord injury, the body's inflammatory cells, among others, produce highly reactive oxidizing agents including "free radicals." Oxidizing agents attack molecules that are crucial for cell function by modifying their chemical structures. This process is called oxidative damage. Oxidative damage occurs in disorders ranging from slow neurodegenerative diseases like amyotrophic lateral sclerosis (ALS or Lou Gehrig's disease) and Parkinson's disease to acute events like stroke and trauma. Thus, it has been the focus of intensive research. Scientists are learning which chemicals are responsible for oxidative damage in the nervous system, how they are generated, and what role the natural antioxidant defense systems play.

Free radicals are produced as a byproduct of normal metabolism. The brain and spinal cord normally have a high rate of oxidative (energy-producing) metabolism. The increases in blood flow during "reperfusion," when blood flow is restored following injury, may raise free radical production even more. Inflammation can also accelerate the production of free radicals. Many scientists believe that superoxides (oxygen molecules with an extra electron) can escape from the normal antioxidant defenses of the CNS and combine with hydrogen peroxide, also normally present, to form hydroxyl radicals (oxygen-hydrogen with an extra electron). In the test tube, hydroxyl radicals are extremely reactive and quickly attack crucial cellular structures and enzymes. However, evidence suggests that this scenario may be different in the living CNS. For one thing, the CNS has concentrations of enzymes that can safely inactivate free radicals. The antioxidant enzyme called copper-zinc superoxide dismutase (SOD), for example, is abundant in the CNS.

Although hydroxyl radicals are the most reactive molecules in the test tube, nitric oxide may be a more important cause of oxidative damage in living animals. Nitric oxide itself is not very destructive -- in fact the body uses it as a signaling molecule -- but it can combine with superoxide ions to produce a very toxic compound called peroxynitrite. Nitric oxide forms peroxynitrite by a reaction that is a million times faster than the one that forms hydroxyl radicals, and it diffuses ten thousand times farther. Peroxynitrite increases its range of damage even more by inactivating some antioxidant defenses, such as SOD. This free radical also can change how cells respond to natural growth and survival factors; for example, it can change the effect of NGF (nerve growth factor) from protecting against apoptosis to accelerating this type of cell death.

The complex actions of nitric oxide illustrate how the interactions between oxidants and biological systems influence how toxic the oxidants' effects can be. These results focus attention on harmful chemical agents that elude antioxidant defenses and attack critical cell molecules. One useful finding is that nitric oxide damage leaves a characteristic molecular "footprint" on cell proteins. This footprint may allow researchers to identify targets of oxidative damage following spinal cord trauma and help in developing therapeutic and protective measures.

Calcium and Excitotoxicity

Following trauma, an excessive release of neurotransmitters - chemical messengers that travel between neurons -- can cause secondary damage by overexciting nerve cells. This phenomenon, called excitotoxicity, has been a major focus of research on stroke and traumatic brain injury, and it may also contribute to neurodegenerative diseases and spinal cord injury. Researchers know about excitotoxicity (and calcium-mediated damage, which often follows) from both cell culture experiments, in which relevant variables are simplified and controlled, and from experiments in the much more complex living animals. Insights about excitotoxicity are now being applied to understanding secondary damage following spinal cord trauma.

Glutamate is the neurotransmitter most often used by nerve cells to activate, or excite, one another.

Excitotoxicity caused by excessive release of glutamate contributes to damage following traumatic CNS injury and stroke. Excessive glutamate can damage nerve cells and glia in several ways. One harmful sequence begins when glutamate overactivates a type of glutamate receptors called NMDA receptors, allowing high levels of calcium to enter the cell. Calcium regulates many cellular processes. For example, calcium activates certain proteases called calpains. Proteases are enzymes that degrade other proteins and have important regulatory roles in cells. Inappropriate activation of these enzymes can damage important parts of the cell. Calcium metabolism is intimately related to oxidative damage as well. Mitochondria--structures within cells that are responsible for producing energy by oxidation -- actively take up calcium. Mitochondria damaged by excessive calcium may produce even more oxidizing free radicals. Excitotoxicity can also damage cells through processes that do not involve calcium. For example, glutamate allows entry into cells of ions such as sodium and chloride that can cause water to enter, leading to uncontrolled swelling.

Necrosis and Apoptosis

New insights about how cells die are dramatically affecting many areas of disease research, and spinal cord injury is no exception. Until recently, scientists believed that necrosis, or uncontrolled cell death, was the only way cells die after CNS trauma. Findings presented at the workshop now suggest that apoptosis (programmed cell death) occurs in parallel with necrosis, and that delayed apoptosis contributes to secondary damage following spinal cord trauma. Cell death programs and experimental interventions to halt them were major themes of the workshop.

Apoptosis occurs in many contexts other than disease. For example, it plays a key role in the developing nervous system. The embryonic spinal cord and brain generate many more neurons than are found in the adult organism. Neurons compete for natural chemicals called trophic factors that are supplied by target cells, and nerve cells that do not make proper connections die by apoptosis.

Many forms of damage can trigger cell death. Cells undergoing apoptosis exhibit changes very different from those of cells dying from necrosis, reflecting the more controlled nature of programmed cell death. Necrotic cells swell and break open, leaking their contents into the surrounding area and provoking an inflammatory response. In apoptosis, cells go through a series of characteristic structural changes. During apoptosis, bubbles or "blebs" form in the outer cell membrane, and membrane-enclosed fragments of the cell may break away. The cell nucleus also condenses and fragments, and polyribosomes (the cellular machinery for synthesizing proteins) break up. In most cells, enzymes cut DNA into unequal pieces. This DNA degradation may have evolved as a defense against viruses that attempt to establish residence within cells. Chemicals released from dying cells then induce surrounding cells to scavenge the debris. Apoptosis eliminates damaged cells without releasing dangerous molecules like proteases and glutamate that might harm neighboring cells.

It is not obvious that preventing apoptosis would be beneficial in spinal cord injury. Cells rescued from apoptosis might go on to die by necrosis and damage their neighbors. Nerve cells that survive a "suicide attempt" might have impaired function and be more disruptive than beneficial. In many cases, necrosis and apoptosis probably occur in parallel. In experiments reported at the workshop, necrosis from excitotoxicity killed most cultured cells from the mouse cerebral cortex. Blocking this excitotoxic necrosis with glutamate antagonist drugs and extending oxygen-glucose deprivation to overcome the protective effect led to apoptosis. Some drugs had opposite effects on necrosis and apoptosis. For example, certain chemical signals promoted necrosis but reduced apoptosis.

Recently, scientists have found that apoptosis contributes to spinal cord cell death and dysfunction after trauma. Necrosis was prominent in rats subjected to severe spinal cord trauma. However, following milder trauma, cells died by apoptosis. Mapping the positions of apoptotic cells within these spinal cords revealed interesting patterns. Apoptosis of nerve cells was largely restricted to sites near the impact zone itself and generally occurred within about 8 hours of the trauma. Apoptosis in glial cells was much more prolonged, and a second wave of apoptosis occurred in the white matter -- probably among oligodendrocytes -- at about 7 days after injury. This wave of secondary death rippled out much further than the original site of injury. In one experiment, moderate-impact contusions in the rat spinal cord caused little apparent structural damage to myelinated axons in the first few hours, but led to extensive demyelination, probably because of delayed apoptosis of oligodendrocytes, by 3 weeks after injury. These results are important in defining the time windows during which therapeutic intervention might be beneficial. Optimal strategies for saving nerve cells may be different from optimal strategies for saving oligodendrocytes.

Much of what we know about the cellular mechanisms that underlie apoptosis comes from studies of the nematode worm C. elegans. This tiny worm has only about 300 nerve cells, each of which is individually recognizable, unlike the uncountable billions of neurons in a mammalian nervous system. These worms also allow genetic manipulations that are much more difficult to perform in mammals. Scientists studying C. elegans have begun to understand the basic elements of the cell death program by observing worms with mutations in genes that control apoptosis. These include death-suppressor genes, killer genes, genes that control engulfment of cell debris, and genes for degrading DNA. Crucial cellular processes are highly conserved in evolution, that is, they don't change much between lower and higher animals. The detection of cell death genes in higher organisms, based on their resemblance to genes in worms, has been key to understanding cell death in mammals.

The best-studied models of mammalian nerve cell apoptosis are cultures of sympathetic nerve cells (a type of PNS cell) from which the critical trophic factor NGF, or nerve growth factor, has been removed. The cell death program initiated by removing NGF includes five stages: activation, propagation, commitment, execution, and death.

Scientists have now defined each stage by cellular events such as the activation of specific genes and enzyme systems. Up until the commitment stage, interrupting the synthesis of new proteins needed for the program to proceed can halt apoptosis. Even after that stage, blocking the actions of certain enzymes, especially a group of protein-degrading enzymes called the ICE (interleukin converting enzyme) family of proteases, can interrupt the death program. Cell death programs may differ among cells; for example, some cells apparently do not require new protein synthesis for apoptosis. Different cell death programs may occur even in the same type of nerve cell in response to different types of injury. In all cases, however, the cells actively participate in the process that leads to their demise.

Using cultured PNS neurons, scientists have tested two strategies for interrupting programmed cell death. One method used drugs that inhibit the ICE family of proteases, proteins that are crucial for the cell death program. The other method used genetically engineered cells lacking bcl-2, a regulator gene needed for the apoptosis program to go forward. In other words, scientists bred mice in which the cell death program was genetically suppressed. Scientists found that regardless of the strategy tested, nerve cells deprived of NGF were arrested in a metabolically quiescent "undead state" for long periods. When subsequently given NGF, these cells were "resurrected" -- they appeared normal and grew.

Similar strategies have been used to block apoptosis in animal models of cerebral ischemia (stroke) and spinal cord injury. In rodent models of stroke, blocking apoptosis, either with drugs or by genetic manipulations, reduced brain damage after blood flow was interrupted. Improved movement in these animals showed that surviving brain cells could still function. Rats with spinal cord injuries that were given an inhibitor of protein synthesis for 1 month were able to retain some use of their hindlimbs. This radical treatment blocked apoptosis by preventing the synthesis of new proteins necessary for the cell death program to go forward.

These studies collectively suggest that blocking cell death programs might buy time that will allow some cells to survive the initial trauma of spinal cord injury. However, the methods used to block cell death in these experiments are not practical for human application: The drugs can be toxic, and genetic manipulation to create humans resistant to injury is obviously not a viable solution. In addition to developing better drugs to block apoptosis, scientists need to answer several key questions about the nature of cell death. These questions include what triggers apoptosis, how developmental apoptosis resembles (or differs from) injury-related apoptosis, how cell death programs and timing vary in different cell types, and to what extent this form of cell death contributes to the functional losses seen in patients with spinal cord injury.

Axon Damage

With the current scientific excitement about cell death, it is important to emphasize that damage to axons causes most of the problems associated with spinal cord injury, including loss of motor control and sensation. In rat spinal cord contusion injuries, for example, recovery of function correlates closely to the number of remaining axons. Until recently, most researchers assumed that the physical forces of spinal cord trauma immediately tear axons. Recent studies of axon damage following traumatic brain injury are changing this view.

Within several days of traumatic brain or spinal cord injury, grossly swollen axons, termed "reactive swellings" or "retraction balls," appear. Many scientists believe that physical forces of trauma stretch axon fibers, causing them to tear and swell. Studies using multiple animal models and various anatomical tracers now have shown that much of the axon damage following CNS trauma is not immediate. Instead, it occurs hours later from swelling caused by impaired axonal transport. Axonal transport is a vital cellular process that moves molecules and cell components from the cell body toward the axon terminal and from the terminal back to the cell body.

What disrupts axonal transport and causes delayed axon damage? There appear to be multiple causes, but changes to the cytoskeleton play a critical role. The cytoskeleton is the internal scaffolding that determines the shapes of cells. It is necessary for transport of substances along the axons. In severe injuries, changes in the cell membrane that surrounds axons can allow an abnormal influx of ions, particularly calcium. This leads to compacting of the cytoskeleton and interruption of axonal transport. Calpain, a calcium-activated protein-degrading enzyme, probably participates in this process. Swelling and disrupted transport also occur in axons whose membranes show no change in ion permeability. In these axons, which predominate in mild to moderate injuries, neurofilaments (one component of the cytoskeleton) become misaligned. This, again, impairs transport and leads to swelling of axons.

Damage to axons has several consequences within the spinal cord. Following axon injury, axons disconnected from their nerve cell bodies disintegrate by a process called "Wallerian" or "orthograde" degeneration. Nerve cell bodies with damaged axons, and the axon segment that remains attached, may die by retrograde degeneration, that is, degeneration that begins at the site of injury and progresses back toward the cell body. From a functional point of view, the delayed death of oligodendrocytes and the resulting demyelination of axons are also critical events, because unmyelinated axons do not conduct electrical impulses normally. The death of these glial cells may result partly from the degeneration of damaged axons because oligodendrocytes apparently require contact with axons to remain healthy. The removal of normal nerve connections also has important consequences. The diverse effects of axon injury suggest that more than one therapeutic approach may be needed to overcome this damage.

Changes below the Injury

While the most dramatic changes in the spinal cord occur at or near the site of injury, the spinal cord also changes below that point. Understanding these changes is becoming more important as researchers learn how to foster axon regeneration.

A key question is what regenerating axons will find when they reach the spinal cord below the injury. Changes below the injury site also influence clinical symptoms, such as reflex changes and spasticity, and they may be a factor in the success of future neural prostheses that might rely upon spinal reflexes or motor control circuits.

The spinal cord is not just a passive conduit carrying signals to and from the brain. It helps to control movement and to interpret sensory information flowing in from the body. Walking, for example, includes three neural processes. First, networks of nerve cells within the spinal cord (central pattern generators) generate the basic motor patterns that activate muscles in the sequence appropriate for walking. Second, sensory feedback from the limbs into the spinal cord modifies this basic motor pattern. Third, control signals from higher centers in the brain modulate the spinal circuits. These higher centers turn the spinal pattern generators on and off, shift between different types of locomotion, control sensory influences according to the type of movements, and govern posture and balance. Scientists are beginning to learn how these systems work and how they come together during development.

How the spinal cord circuitry below the trauma site changes following injury is poorly understood, but scientists are beginning to recognize that these changes are important. In one series of experiments, scientists transected the spinal cords of chick embryos and removed a segment. Spinal cords in very young chick embryos regenerated remarkably well. In older embryos, however, axons did not regenerate and many motor neurons, interneurons, and sensory neurons died below the injury. This cell death resulted from the injury rather than from the programmed cell death that normally occurs during development. These experiments suggest that death of cells below the site of injury may be a factor in human spinal cord injury as well.

Spinal cord injury also may alter connections among nerve cells that survive below the injury. The adult CNS is much more plastic, or changeable, than scientists believed just a few years ago. One interesting discovery is that some of the cellular mechanisms that allow the nervous system to adapt with experience, such as glutamate signaling and calcium-mediated events, are the same as those that go awry after injury and cause secondary damage. This discovery may explain why some of these apparently harmful mechanisms have persisted in evolution.

Immediately after spinal cord trauma, nerve cells below the site of injury are excited by trauma-induced release of neurotransmitters. A loss of normal excitatory and inhibitory signals follows when the severed axons die. In many parts of the CNS, including the spinal cord, strong excitation of neurons modifies the strength of synapses. This form of plasticity might alter the remaining circuits of the spinal cord in unpredictable ways. The removal of normal signals also provokes sprouting of nearby axons into the territory vacated by degenerating axons. The consequences of this rewiring are hard to predict. They may include the changes in reflexes often seen in people with spinal cord injury. These complex and diverse consequences suggest that attention to the changes below the site of spinal cord injury may be essential for successful regeneration and rehabilitation.

Conclusion

Scientists who have been studying spinal cord injury for many years say that spinal cord injury research has now come of age. Because of progress in neuroscience, as well as in spinal cord injury research, researchers can test specific ideas about how changes in cells and molecules affect spinal cord injury. Not long ago, only descriptive studies were possible. Oxidative free radicals, calcium-mediated damage, proteases, cytoskeletal dysfunction, excitotoxicity, immune reactions, apoptosis, and necrosis all come into play following spinal cord injury. These sources of secondary damage interact in complex ways that scientists are just beginning to understand. What is encouraging is that each of these harmful processes offers targets for developing therapies.

Much of the workshop discussion about secondary injury processes relied upon experiments in fields other than spinal cord injury, especially stroke and traumatic brain injury. The potential for application of such findings to spinal cord injury was one of the most exciting aspects of the workshop. While scientists do not agree about how directly this information will apply to the specifics of spinal cord trauma, most believe that studying other disorders can provide insights that will improve understanding of spinal cord injury. Most importantly, studies in other experimental systems can provide hypotheses to test in models of spinal cord injury.

Chapter 6

Regeneration

For successful regeneration to occur following spinal cord injury, several things must happen. First, damaged nerve cells and supporting cells must survive or be replaced, despite the acute effects of trauma and the conspiracy of processes that cause secondary damage. Replacement of lost cells in the CNS is unlikely without intervention because adult nerve cells in the brain and spinal cord cannot divide. Nerve cells that survive the injury often must regrow axons, despite tissue changes such as cavity formation that obstruct growth. Axons also must navigate among the myriad possibilities to find appropriate targets. Once the axons locate their targets, they must construct specialized structures to release neurotransmitters at synapses, while target cells must assemble and precisely locate the structures needed to respond to neurotransmitters. Finally, the neural circuitry may have to compensate for changes that have occurred in the spinal cord circuitry following injury.

Until recently, most scientists believed that nerve cells in the CNS of adult mammals could not regenerate. Dramatic findings, some presented at this workshop, are now changing that pessimistic outlook. For example, some studies have demonstrated that nerve cells in the brain and spinal cord make unsuccessful attempts to regenerate and can regrow under some conditions. New findings also demonstrate that the spinal cord has more active repair mechanisms than previously suspected. Although researchers recognize the many obstacles to obtaining regeneration in the human spinal cord, they believe successful regeneration of even a small percentage of nerve fibers will produce significant recovery of function.

Implications of Development

Scientists favor the spinal cord for studying the CNS because it is simpler than the brain. The long tradition of anatomical and physiological research on the cord provides a solid framework for studying development. Developing nerve cells perform the same steps needed for regeneration -- they grow, navigate, and make appropriate connections. Regenerating nerve fibers face problems that are quite different from those faced by developing nerve cells, however. For example, the tissue through which axons move is more loosely connected during development, and an injured spinal cord may become quite disorganized near the injury site. Also, distances in the adult CNS are much greater than in the embryo, and chemical signposts for navigating axons may have changed in the adult. While the extent to which regeneration resembles development is uncertain, research about nervous system development is a source of crucial insights about how to promote regeneration following spinal cord injury.

Nerve Cell Differentiation

The adult spinal cord is an intricate assembly of cells and nerve fibers arrayed in specific locations with very precise interconnections. Nerve cells in the spinal cord include several types of motor neurons, sensory neurons, and interneurons, each of which varies in shape, electrical activity, neurotransmitter release, and many aspects. Glial cells also include several specialized types of cells in the mature CNS, and the major nerve pathways of the spinal cord white matter are highly organized anatomically. How all of this comes about has been a subject of speculation and experiments for more than a century. The mystery is finally giving way to traditional neuroscience research methods, augmented by new technologies such as molecular genetics.

The factors causing cell types in the spinal cord to become distinct from one another are cell lineage (which cells arise from which by cell division) and cues from within the developing embryo. Research is now identifying these chemical cues and discovering how cells respond to them. Two major signaling systems control the fate of embryonic brain and spinal cord cells. One system controls the specialization of the nervous system along the long axis from the brain down through the spinal cord. The other system controls specialization along the dorsoventral plane, that is, in a cross-section of the spinal cord ("dorsal" refers to the back portion and "ventral" denotes the abdominal direction). So far, the general operating principles of the two systems appear to be the same.

The control of cell identity along the dorsoventral axis of the spinal cord illustrates how these developmental systems operate. Among the essential tools scientists developed to study this process are chemical markers that stain specific cell types before they fully specialize in the embryonic spinal cord. Three cell types form in the ventral part of the early embryonic spinal cord. Glial cells form in the most ventral part, called the floor plate; motor neurons and interneurons form more dorsally. Experiments have shown that the key signal that determines the fate of all three cell types is a protein called sonic hedgehog. (The name arises because this mammalian molecule was identified by its resemblance to the "hedgehog" protein of the fruitfly. Flies with a mutation in the hedgehog gene have a peculiar prickly appearance.) To simulate the situation in the developing embryo, scientists placed pieces of ventral spinal cord in cell culture and exposed them to different concentrations of sonic hedgehog protein. These pieces produced motor neurons, glia, or interneurons depending on the concentration of protein to which they were exposed. In the embryo, a structure called the notochord releases the sonic hedgehog protein signal. Spinal cord cells that lie closest to the notochord are exposed to the highest concentration of the signal and become glial cells. Those in more dorsal positions are exposed to lesser concentrations and become, respectively, motor neurons and interneurons.

Although scientists are rapidly identifying the signals that drive the generation of cell types in the developing spinal cord, many basic questions remain. Many signals have yet to be discovered, and it is not yet clear how cells sense small differences in concentrations and respond to become specialized cell types. Interactions among the various signaling systems are likewise obscure.

Answers to these questions may have implications for spinal cord regeneration. In the last few years, scientists have discovered that even the mature CNS may harbor latent progenitor cells that can divide and specialize to form new nerve and glial cells. In a rat model of spinal cord trauma, the single layer of cells lining the central canal of the spinal cord expands to multiple layers of cells about 48 hours after a contusion lesion. The central canal is continuous with the brain ventricles, large fluid-filled spaces inside the brain. During development, new nerve cells arise from cells lining these structures. Cells from the expanded central canal of injured animals appear to stream out into the spinal cord; these may be neural progenitor cells attempting to repair damaged tissue. It is important to know whether developmental signals that might guide neuron growth persist in the adult. Another reason studies of cell specialization may be relevant to spinal cord injury is that the molecules involved in this developmental process may have other important functions in the adult. Understanding the signals that control cell specialization in development may be critical for learning how to help them repair damaged spinal cords.

Many new findings presented at the workshop reflected the ways researchers now study the molecular machinery by which cells operate. Knowing the genetic code for proteins allows scientists to detect similarities among proteins. By comparing genes among different species, researchers can rapidly apply insights from lower organisms to mammals. Comparing newly identified genes and proteins to known ones within the same animal can also help scientists understand what a newly discovered protein does. Identifying one protein often helps reveal other members of the same protein family that have related functions, as in families of growth factors, cell adhesion molecules, and neurotransmitter receptors. Scientists are also learning to recognize functional regions that many proteins share in different combinations. Gene sequences predict many aspects of a protein's function, such as whether it will respond to certain regulator molecules. Thus, the chemical language that orchestrates development provides crucial clues about regeneration, even if the processes differ.

Axon Path finding

Developing nerve cells of the brain and spinal cord grow axons over long distances, along specific routes, and to precise targets. The tip of a growing axon forms a specialized structure called a growth cone. These growth cones sense cues, integrate that information, and make choices that steer the axon in one direction or another. Scientists have identified attractants and repellents that diffuse over long distances, as well as chemical attractants and repellents with fixed locations. Together, these cues allow axons to navigate through the developing brain and spinal cord. The identification of one family of long-distance attractants, the netrins, illustrates this area of research and its potential relevance to spinal cord regeneration.

A century ago, the Spanish neuroanatomist Ramón y Cajal speculated that diffusible chemical signals might guide growing axons. The first such signals, called netrins, were discovered just a few years ago in the chick spinal cord. "Commissural" neurons in the dorsal part of the spinal cord send axons from the front of the cord around toward the back. When the growth cones of these axons approach the midline of the developing spinal cord, they make a beeline for the floor plate, a specialized region of the embryonic spinal cord at the ventral edge of the midline. When scientists placed pieces of developing spinal cords in various arrangements in culture, they found that something in the ventral floorplate attracted growing commissural axons from a distance.

They isolated the attractants and named the identified proteins netrins. When scientists further examined the effects of netrins, they found that these molecules also repelled growing axons from other types of developing nerve cells. This finding was predicted by studies in worms of molecules that closely resemble netrins. Experiments in normal and mutant mice confirmed that these molecules guide developing axons in living mammals. **(source:** *www.ninds.nih.gov › News From NINDS › Proceedings)*

Many guidance molecules were only recently identified, and certainly more remain to be found. Similarities between guidance molecules in mammals and those in simple organisms like worms and fruitflies are speeding progress in this area of neurobiology. Whether regenerating axons respond to guidance signals in the same manner as developing axons and whether these cues are still present in the adult spinal cord are particularly important questions for spinal cord regeneration. Ultimately, scientists hope to find ways to manipulate these signaling mechanisms to enhance regeneration.

Synapse Formation

For regeneration to be successful, axons must not only grow but also find and connect to appropriate targets. Axons must construct the highly specialized structures that release neurotransmitters from nerve terminals. Cells that receive signals across synapses also must participate in forming new synapses at a time when they would not normally do so. They must assemble in precisely the right places the specialized structures necessary to respond to neurotransmitters. Finally, the developing spinal cord must insure that synapses of the correct type form only on proper cells and on the appropriate parts of these cells so that the neural circuits will work.

Although scientists know very little about how new synapses form in the adult mammalian spinal cord, they are learning how synapses develop in the skeletal neuromuscular junctions (NMJs), the synapses by which motor neurons activate muscle cells. NMJs are much more accessible for study than synapses in the spinal cord, and scientists have therefore used them to learn about the basic principles of synapse development and function. These nerve-muscle synapses also regenerate, which allows comparison of development and regeneration.

Although axons and muscle cells can each synthesize the specialized components they need to form synapses, development of synapses requires back-and-forth signaling between the two cell types. At the turn of the century, scientists demonstrated that regenerating motor nerves form synapses at the exact sites of former synapses, even though synapses cover only a tiny percentage of the available muscle surface. This means muscle cells must have "stop signals" that axons can recognize. Muscles also regulate their receptivity to synapse formation according to whether they already have a nerve connection. An implanted nerve will not form a synapse with a muscle unless the original nerve to that muscle has been removed. Muscles that have lost their nerve connections may also release molecules that entice axons to make new synapses.

In the modern era, scientists have added the tools of genetics to traditional methods of developmental neuroscience research. They can now test the role of particular molecules in synapse formation by creating mutant mice, such as "knockout mice," that lack a particular protein. Studies with knockout mice have shown how a protein called agrin helps the developing muscle aggregate molecules called acetylcholine receptors at the synapse where they are needed. Acetylcholine receptors enable muscle cells to respond to the neurotransmitter acetylcholine, which is released from the nerve terminal. Agrin knockout mice died before birth or were stillborn because of defective NMJs. Interestingly, inactivating the agrin gene not only affected muscle, but also the perturbed axons. This reflects the complex interactive nature of the signaling process between axons and their targets, which scientists are just beginning to understand. Scientists are now creating genetically altered mice to study other molecules that control the development of the NMJ.

In many ways, synapses within the brain and spinal cord resemble the NMJ, but not completely. Some, but not all, of the molecules that control development of the NMJ are present in the developing CNS. Each muscle cell receives synapses from only one axon, and all of these use the same neurotransmitter (acetylcholine). A single spinal cord nerve cell, on the other hand, may receive thousands of synapses from nerve cells of the brain and spinal cord and from sensory nerves of the body. Each spinal cord neuron may also respond to several different neurotransmitters. So, while spinal cord synapses and NMJ probably share the same general principles, the spinal cord must need additional signals to form synapses.

Understanding synapse formation is becoming increasingly important as the prospect improves for obtaining survival and growth of spinal cord cells after injury. So far, nerve fibers regrowing in experimental animal models of spinal cord regeneration have developed few new synapses, and this may be the limiting factor in recovery of movement. Understanding how synapses develop may reveal whether spinal regeneration stops because regenerating axons lack the ability to form synapses or whether nerve cells below the lesion are unreceptive to synapse formation. This may lead to ways of encouraging the formation of new synapses by regenerating fibers.

Basic Regeneration Studies

Scientists have long known that nerve cells outside the brain and spinal cord can regenerate, but they believed that nerve cells in the CNS of adults could not regrow. In the early 1980s, experiments in the spinal cords of animals showed that CNS neurons can regrow under certain conditions. These experiments were inspired by the idea that adult CNS cells might be able to grow if given a permissive growth environment. Scientists grafted segments of sciatic nerve -- a peripheral nerve that can regenerate -- to the spinal cord, circumventing the lesion site. Some nerve cells, usually from near the site of the lesion, grew axons through the nerve bridges as far as 3 or 4 centimeters and reached the other end of the bridge. Some nerve cells in the lower parts of the brain also grew into the graft. Because of the complexity of the spinal cord, researchers could not accurately assess whether regrowing nerve cells made functional synapses or exactly what about the sciatic nerve bridges was "permissive." For this reason, some scientists turned to another model system to study CNS regeneration--the retina.

The retina of the eye is an outpost of the brain. Like the spinal cord, it is part of the CNS. Retinal neurons called ganglion cells carry signals from the retina to the brain. Their axons, together with supporting cells, form the optic nerve. Cutting or crushing the optic nerve, and thus the axons of the retinal ganglion cells, has become an important model for injury and regeneration in the CNS.

Retinal ganglion cells normally do not regenerate after the optic nerve has been transected. In early experiments, scientists placed peripheral nerve bridges from the site of damage in optic nerves (usually near the retina) to appropriate targets in the brain. The nerve grafts bypassed the problem of pathfinding by funneling growing axons directly to the correct region of the brain. Some ganglion cell axons grew distances equivalent to nearly twice their normal length. However, at best only a small percentage of axons regrew in these experiments since most cells died soon after transection. Some axons did penetrate the brain and make synapses, restoring the simple reflex response of pupils to light and the animals' light-avoidance behavior.

Axons that reached the brain found the appropriate layers and parts of cells in the brain, but failed to recreate the proper, orderly representation of the visual world on the brain.

These retinal regeneration experiments raised many questions. What makes peripheral nervous system tissue supportive for growth? Are there growth factors in the nerve grafts that are not available in the adult CNS, or are growth inhibitors normally present in the adult CNS absent from the grafts? Why do so many ganglion cells die and so few regenerate? Do intrinsic genetic programs of these cells affect success and failure? How does regeneration resemble and differ from development?

Experiments are beginning to answer these kinds of questions.

Trophic Factors

For nerve cells to regenerate axons, they must first survive the injury. Trophic factors are signals that promote the survival and growth of nerve cells. The classical studies of trophic factors in development showed that nerve cells become dependent on these substances during the period when they specialize and begin to connect with their targets. The developing nervous system produces many more nerve cells than the adult nervous system needs. Cells compete with one another to obtain trophic factors supplied by appropriate target cells. Those neurons that do not succeed in competing for appropriate connections die through apoptosis.

The first trophic factor isolated was NGF (nerve growth factor). NGF is essential for the survival of some types of nerve cells in the PNS. Withdrawing NGF from peripheral neurons in culture is an important way of studying apoptosis in nerve cells. In the last several years, scientists have found that trophic factors are important in the development of the CNS as well. At the workshop, participants reported experiments suggesting that there are important differences in the trophic factor requirements of central and peripheral nerve cells. Those differences may help explain why CNS nerve cells do not regenerate.

Here again, retinal ganglion cells are favorable subjects for CNS research. Scientists developed methods to isolate these cells with 99 percent purity, allowing precise studies of the factors these cells need to survive and grow. The scientists then attempted to sustain these cells in culture using trophic factors that the cells might encounter in their normal course from the retina to the brain. None of these factors alone was sufficient for more than 1 percent of retinal ganglion cells to survive for even 3 days.

Studies in peripheral nerve cells have shown that activating the cyclic AMP "second messenger" system augments the effects of trophic factors. Cyclic AMP is a small molecule that carries messages from cell surface receptors activated by "first messengers" (hormones, neurotransmitters, or other signals) to sites within the cell. Like other second messenger systems, this biochemical pathway allows a single first messenger to control several cellular processes and helps in regulating and integrating the many signals cells receive. Although activating the cyclic AMP second messenger pathway with the drug forskolin did not sustain retinal ganglion cells in culture, and trophic factors alone were insufficient, the two combined saved more than a third of the cultured cells. Combining multiple trophic factors with forskolin allowed survival of more than half of the cultured cells for more than a month.

Adding other, as yet unpurified, factors boosted survival to more than 80 percent.

These experiments suggest that combinations of trophic factors may be essential for survival of CNS neurons. Another important insight is that the responsiveness of CNS cells to trophic factors is not static, but can change depending on the level of second messengers. Electrical activity and signals from other cells stimulate second messenger systems, and these influences change dramatically for cells below a spinal cord injury. Administering trophic factors and controlling responsiveness to these factors may promote nerve cell survival in the damaged spinal cord. However, these powerful and poorly understood substances can also have serious side effects.

Scientists are not yet certain whether adult spinal cord nerve cells need combinations of trophic factors, which trophic factors affect which cell types, or what controls the cells' sensitivity to these factors. In one important finding from the retina culture experiments, scientists learned that survival and axon growth were always coupled; that is, any interventions that allowed cells to survive also prompted them to extend their axons.

Intrinsic Growth Programs

Nerve cells' intrinsic capacity to grow is another factor that may contribute to the success or failure of regeneration. Scientists have studied intrinsic growth capacity by comparing cells from young animals to those from older ones. Very young animals generally recover more completely from CNS damage than do adult animals. By placing the retina and the tectum (the brain area to which retinal ganglion cells connect) from animals together in culture, scientists demonstrated that regeneration in culture is also age-dependent. They then independently varied the age of the tectal and retinal pieces placed together in culture to determine to what extent each contributed to the failure to grow in older animals. The results showed two major reductions in the ability of ganglion cells to grow as the animal ages. The first, larger reduction was due to changes in the growth capacity of the retinal cells themselves. The later, smaller reduction, was more gradual and appeared to be due mostly to changes in the target tissue. Providing growth factors partially increased survival and growth but could not overcome the early large decline in growth ability.

Biologists believe changes in growth capacity probably reflect changes in the specific genes that are active in each cell. Several genes were inactivated at about the time that regeneration declined, but one gene was turned off just as the capacity to regenerate was lost. Surprisingly, that gene was bcl-2, which is well-known because its product is an important regulator of apoptosis. Retinal ganglion cells taken from mice with an inactivated bcl-2 gene (bcl-2 knockout mice) did not show the normal sharp decline in growth ability. Even cells from the adult retina of these knockout mice could grow if they were given embryonic tissue as a target. Experiments with drugs directed at enzymes in the apoptosis pathway showed that the bcl-2 gene's effects on growth were separate from its effects on apoptosis. This gene apparently acts as a "switch" that controls axon growth in the CNS. Finding ways to control this switch may yield a new approach to therapy for spinal cord injury that may complement other therapies such as trophic factors. While this treatment approach appears beyond genetic technology at the moment, understanding the role played by these intrinsic programs in regulating the neuron growth will provide important insights into regeneration.

Barriers to Growth

Scientists have now identified a long list of molecules in the adult CNS that actively inhibit growth. For example, oligodendrocytes produce a myelin-associated growth inhibitor that may be one of the most important inhibitors of growth in the adult spinal cord. One way these inhibitors act is by making growth cones collapse. Growth inhibition may be quite specific for each nerve cell type; that is, different cells may be most sensitive to different inhibitors. Another way inhibitors act is by modifying the extracellular matrix, the noncellular material surrounding cells through which axons must grow. For example, some substances act as "anti-adhesives," preventing growing axons from sticking to surrounding tissue, which is necessary for them to grow forward. How inhibitors block axon growth and which of the many inhibitors are clinically important following spinal cord injury are essential questions that scientists are now trying to answer.

Scientists need to determine the normal physiological roles of the many substances that inhibit growth in the adult spinal cord. Similarities in how these inhibitors work might allow generic strategies for overcoming their effects. One possibility would be to find common pathways, such as second messenger systems, through which these factors operate. Experiments with a component of pertussis toxin (a toxin from the bacteria that causes whooping cough) suggest that this might be possible. This toxin, which affects second messengers, blocked growth cone collapse from three very different inhibitory factors (collapsin-1, thrombin, and the myelin-associated factor). Because the extracellular matrix that surrounds cells is a repository for many inhibitory substances, understanding the interaction of cells with the extracellular matrix is an important focus of research. Finally, signals that inhibit and stimulate growth might converge on common intracellular machinery so that sufficient stimulation might overcome some of the inhibition. Experiments with trophic factors in retinal ganglion cells support this idea.

Applied Regeneration Studies

Researchers are beginning to apply knowledge about nerve growth and inhibitory factors and other aspects of neuron regeneration by testing new therapeutic approaches in animal models of spinal cord injury. The partial success of several of these animal experiments has led to optimism by many experts that, with the right combination of strategies, regeneration will eventually become possible in humans. However, it now appears unlikely that there will be a single magic bullet for repairing the spinal cord. Instead, a combination of approaches will probably be necessary.

Transplantation

One approach for repairing spinal cords that is being tested in animals is to transplant cells and tissues into the damaged spinal cord. In particular, scientists are transplanting cells or pieces of peripheral nerves that produce substances that create an environment for axons to grow. This idea was first advocated about 100 years ago by the neurologist Ramón y Cajal. He suggested implanting cells from the PNS into the area of a CNS injury. Since the environment of the PNS supports axon regeneration, he believed re-creating this environment in the spinal cord might allow CNS axons to regrow after an injury. Ideally, this environment would also point growing nerves to the correct targets. Experiments with PNS transplants in rat models of spinal cord injury have led to axon elongation and cell body changes associated with regrowth. Transplants from the PNS also seem to reduce scarring around the injury that may impede regrowth. One technique tested in rats is transplanting Schwann cells -- glial cells that help myelinate axons in the PNS -- into the spinal cord after injury. These transplants supported regrowth of the damaged nerves in rats with spinal cord injury. Researchers are now studying human Schwann cells to determine if this technique will work in humans.

Another way of encouraging regeneration is to implant fetal tissue. Tissue from a growing fetus contains stem cells, progenitor cells, and many substances that support growth. Such tissue also presents fewer obstacles to growing axons. Stem cells can differentiate into several cell types, depending on the signals they receive. Transplanting them into the spinal cord may, with the right chemical signals, help them develop into neurons and supporting cells in the spinal cord, re-establishing lost circuits.

Studies in rats show that fetal transplants promote survival and regrowth of some damaged nerve cells. Transplanting fetal CNS tissue into the spinal cord of both mature and newborn rats yielded axon growth that terminated within a few millimeters of the border of the transplant. Researchers still need to learn exactly how fetal tissue transplants promote nerve regrowth. The transplants appear to "rescue" axons and provide a bridge across which regenerating axons can grow. While both adult and newborn rats regrew descending nerve fibers from the brain, the growth of descending pathways into the transplants was substantially greater in the newborns. This suggests that other changes in the maturing CNS, such as the production of inhibitory factors or a loss of certain axon guidance molecules, may influence axonal regrowth after injury.

Trophic Factors

Using insights from retina and culture experiments, researchers are beginning to test whether trophic factors can enhance regrowth in the spinal cords of rats. Growth factors may be responsible for much of the nerve regeneration normally seen in the PNS and in CNS axons near transplanted PNS tissue.

Different pathways in the spinal cord may require particular combinations of growth factors for survival after injury. While nerve cells usually do not survive after axons have been severed close to the cell body, recent experiments in the rat spinal cord have shown that two trophic factors, brain-derived neurotrophic factor (BDNF) and neurotrophin 3 (NT3), can rescue nerve cells from which the axons have been recently severed. Although NT3 has short-term effects, BDNF can help nerve cells survive for 4 weeks or more after injury. When the trophic factors BDNF, NT3, and NT4 (neurotrophin 4) were combined with fetal tissue transplants, axons no longer stopped growing at the border of the transplant but instead greatly expanded the territory into which they projected.

The combination of transplants and trophic factors also led to an increase in c-jun, an important immediate early gene. Immediate early genes respond rapidly to many stimuli and regulate many cell functions. Interestingly, these experiments showed that axons from cells that use the neurotransmitter serotonin responded to trophic factors more vigorously than axons from cells that use other neurotransmitters. This illustrates the importance of finding the right combination of growth factors for each type of cell.

Anti-Inhibitory Factors

Myelin-associated neurite growth inhibitor, which is produced by oligodendrocytes, is the most important CNS growth inhibitor so far identified. When researchers blocked this growth inhibitor with an antibody called IN-1, which binds to and masks the factor from growth cones, severed axons began extending past the oligodendrocytes and reconnecting with their targets. After this treatment, rats with severed spinal cords moved more normally and partially regained their contact-placing reflexes (in which rats move their legs to support their bodies when they are placed against a surface).

Combination Therapies

Evidence that combining some therapies may have an additive effect has prompted researchers to focus effort on finding a combination that will achieve regeneration. Some combination therapies recently tested in rats have shown exciting results. One approach used neurotrophin 3, fetal cell transplants, and IN-1, the antibody to myelin-associated neurite growth inhibitor. Rats treated with this approach showed faster and more extensive recovery after spinal cord injury than those given any single treatment alone. Their recovered reflexes disappeared after researchers destroyed the cerebral cortex, showing that the brain, rather than reorganization within the spinal cord, controlled the reflexes. Researchers still need to learn if this therapy can be a general approach or if specific nerve pathways have specific requirements for growth. They also need to carefully define the time windows for effective combination treatment.

Another approach using nerve fiber transplantation combined with growth factors showed the first functional regeneration of completely transected rat spinal cords. Researchers carefully transplanted 18 pieces of peripheral nerves (one to three pieces for each of the normal nerve tracts) taken from the rats' chests to "bridge" 5-millimeter gaps at the T8 segment of rats' spinal cords. To evade inhibitory proteins from oligodendrocytes, the bridges routed regenerating axons away from white matter, where they would normally grow, and into gray matter. The researchers fixed the grafts in place with a glue based on a blood-clotting factor called fibrin. The glue also contained acidic fibroblastic growth factor, or aFGF, which enhances nerve fiber development. Finally, the scientists wired the vertebrae to keep the spine in place while the area healed.

After 3 weeks, rats that had received this type of graft began to recover function in their hind legs. Some of the treated rats regained some movement on both sides of their bodies, while others regained movement on only one side. The rats that recovered on both sides of their bodies eventually began partially supporting their weight with their hind limbs. They also displayed walking movements and contact-placing reflexes. The rats continued to improve gradually over the course of a year, though they never walked normally. Rats with bridges from white matter to other white matter, rats in which the fibrin glue had no aFGF, and rats that did not receive transplants did not recover any function over time.

Anatomical studies of spinal cords from rats that recovered function after this therapy showed that the nerve fibers grew into the gray matter on the opposite side of the gap. The fibers then grew at the interface between the gray matter and the white matter, an area that corresponds to the normal corticospinal tract in rats. The degree of recovery corresponded significantly to the degree of motor fiber regeneration.

Conclusion

Basic research has led to a better understanding of trophic factors, growth barriers in the CNS, and the intrinsic capacity of nerve cells to grow. These insights are being applied in animal models of spinal cord injury using transplantation, trophic factors, and anti-inhibitory molecules. The exciting results of strategies that combine these interventions suggest that such approaches will ultimately prove the most successful for regenerating spinal cord pathways in humans. Developmental studies of cell specialization, axon growth and pathfinding, and synapse formation are leading to promising new avenues for improving on these combination approaches.

Chapter 7

Management Principles of Spinal Cord Injuries

Current Interventions

While the possibilities for new therapies deserve much attention, research also may be able to improve existing strategies, including drug therapy, neural prostheses, and rehabilitation.

Drug Therapy

Effective drug therapy for spinal cord injury first became a reality in 1990, when methylprednisolone, the first drug shown to improve recovery from spinal cord injury, moved from clinical trials to standard use. The NASCIS II (National Acute Spinal Cord Injury Study II) trial, a multicenter clinical trial comparing methylprednisolone to placebo and to the drug naloxone, showed that methylprednisolone given within 8 hours after injury significantly improves recovery in humans. Completely paralyzed patients given methylprednisolone recovered an average of about 20 percent of their lost motor function, compared to 8 percent recovery of function in untreated patients. Paretic (partially paralyzed) patients recovered an average of 75 percent of their function, compared to 59 percent in people who did not receive the drug. Patients treated with naloxone, or treated with methylprednisolone more than 8 hours after injury, did not improve significantly more than patients given a placebo.

The successful clinical trial of methylprednisolone revolutionized thinking in the medical community. The trial showed conclusively that there is a window of opportunity for acute treatment of spinal cord injury. Some doctors are now using this idea to guide surgical treatment as well as drug therapy. Today, most patients with spinal cord injuries receive methylprednisolone within 3 hours after injury, especially if the injury is severe. This shows that emergency rooms and acute care facilities are aware of the drug's value and are capable of providing rapid treatment for spinal cord trauma. Success in delivering this drug on a widespread basis shows that health care systems are capable of providing rapid treatment. The NASCIS II trial also proves that well-designed trials of acute therapies for spinal cord injury are feasible and provides a model for testing other interventions.

Other drugs are now being tested in clinical trials. A recently completed trial suggested that 48-hour regimen of methylprednisolone may be warranted in some patients. Preliminary clinical trials of another agent, GM-1 ganglioside, have shown that it is useful in preventing secondary damage in acute spinal cord injury, and other studies suggest that it may also improve neurological recovery from spinal cord injury during rehabilitation.

Neural Prostheses

While it may eventually become possible to help injured spinal cords regrow their connections, another approach is to compensate for lost function by using neural prostheses to circumvent the damage. These sophisticated electrical and mechanical devices connect with the nervous system to supplement or replace lost motor and sensory functions. Neural prostheses for deafness, known as cochlear implants, are now in widespread use in humans and have had a dramatic impact on the lives of some people. The first prostheses for spinal cord injured patients are now being tested in humans. One device, a neural prosthesis that allows rudimentary hand control, was recently approved by the United States Food and Drug Administration (FDA). This prosthesis has been experimentally implanted in more than 60 people. Patients control the device using shoulder muscles. With training, most patients with this device can open and close their hand in two different grasping movements and lock the grasp in place by moving their shoulder in different ways. These simple movements allow the patients to perform many activities of daily life that they would otherwise be unable to perform, such as using silverware, pouring a drink, answering a telephone, and writing a note.

Neural prostheses are complex and contain many intricate components, such as implantable stimulators, electrodes, leads and connectors, sensors, and programming systems. There are many technical considerations in selecting each component. The electronic components must be as small as possible. Biocompatibility between electrodes and body tissue is also necessary to prevent the person from being harmed by contact with the device and to prevent the device from being harmed by contact with the person. Other challenges include finding ways to safely send currents into the body, to reliably record neural activity, and to cope with changes in muscle properties due to the injury. Neural prostheses also must be evaluated for usefulness and long-term safety.

Although many years of intensive study have contributed to the development of the prostheses now being tested, they are really the first generation of useful devices. Better materials and enhanced technology can refine these devices to provide much better function. Among the recent technical advances are extremely small probes that fit 16 electrodes on a shaft finer than a human hair. Integrated into a neural prosthesis, this type of electrode could provide extremely selective stimulation within the CNS, allowing the patient much more refined muscle control and a greater range of function. Future clinical development may allow easier, faster, and more natural movements; improve the longevity and reliability of components; and eliminate external cabling systems and external mounting of sensors.

Further research to improve components and increase understanding of brain circuits may yield prostheses that can provide sensory information to the brain. This will improve both the safety of the devices and the patient's performance of tasks. Devices now being developed may eventually enable people with spinal cord injury to stand unassisted and to use signals from the brain, instead of muscles, to control movement. Other types of neural prostheses currently being developed around the world aim to improve respiratory functions, bladder control, and fecal continence. Ultimately, researchers may be able to harness reflexes or the innate pattern-generating abilities of the spinal cord's central pattern generators to help people with spinal cord injuries walk.

Rehabilitation

Rehabilitation techniques can greatly improve patients' health and quality of life by helping them learn to use their remaining abilities. Studies of problems that spinal cord injury patients experience, such as spasticity, muscle weakness, and impaired motor coordination, are leading to new strategies that may overcome these challenges. As they gain a better understanding of what causes these problems, physicians are learning how to treat them, sometimes using drugs already available for other health problems.

Spasticity, in which abnormal stretch reflexes intensify muscle resistance to passive movements, often develops after spinal cord injury. Several factors may contribute to spasticity. Changes in the strength of connections between neurons or in the neurons themselves may alter the threshold of the stretch reflex. Spinal cord injury also may release one type of interneurons from control by a class of neurotransmitters that includes serotonin and norepinephrine. This change in the balance of neurotransmitters may increase these neurons' excitability and enhance stretch reflexes. Drugs that mimic serotonin can partially restore reflexes, a finding that supports this neurotransmitter theory. Another possible cause of spasticity is that the reactions of pressure receptors in the skin may become stronger, causing muscle spasms that may grow stronger with time. Interneurons activated by NMDA receptors also may contribute to spasticity. NMDA receptors probably help adjust the strength of connections in the brain during learning. Researchers have found that a class of drugs that blocks NMDA receptors can restore stretch reflexes to almost normal strength.

The muscle weakness that frequently occurs after spinal cord injury may result from a loss of excitatory signals from the descending tracts. Abnormal patterns of motor activation in muscles may also contribute by making muscles less efficient so that they tire more easily. Loss of serotonin and related neurotransmitters may disrupt the process that controls how much each nerve cell's activity increases with increasingly strong stimuli. Restoring normal neurotransmitter signals with drugs may partially relieve these problems. Some muscle weakness may also result from abnormal patterns of muscle usage or from changes in muscle properties, including muscular atrophy and growth of connective tissue.

Scientists believe another common motor problem, muscle incoordination, may result in part from the substantial brain reorganization that occurs after injury to the CNS. With a better understanding of how the spinal cord changes following injury, researchers may be able to use drugs or physical therapy to promote reorganization when it is useful and block it when it is harmful.

Rehabilitation strategies will continue to play an important role in the management of spinal cord injury, and they will increase in importance as the ultimate goal of functional spinal cord regeneration is realized. Studies in animals with spinal cord injuries have shown that recovery of movement is linked to the type of training the animals receive. Physical therapy and other rehabilitation strategies also are crucial for maintaining flexibility and muscle strength and for reorganizing the nervous system. These factors will be vital to recovering movement following regeneration as well as maximizing the use of undamaged nerve fibers.

PRECLINICAL AND CLINICAL TESTING OF NEW THERAPIES

Researchers have identified a wide variety of potential therapies for spinal cord injury. To efficiently evaluate these therapies, however, investigators need to carry out well-designed preclinical and clinical trials that will reveal the benefits and drawbacks of each strategy.

Preclinical Testing

Each of the factors contributing to secondary damage presents opportunities for therapeutic intervention. Among these are neuroprotective drugs that might be combined with or even replace methylprednisolone. These drugs include antioxidants, calcium blockers, and drugs that control excitotoxicity. Drugs that enhance axon signaling, such as 4-aminopyridine, form another category of potential therapies. Drugs designed to promote regeneration by capitalizing on newfound knowledge about guidance molecules, trophic factors, and growth-inhibiting substances make up a third class. Other kinds of interventions, such as transplantation, peripheral nerve grafts, hypothermia (cooling), and combinations of therapies also show promise in regrowing spinal cord tracts and promoting recovery of function.

While all of these potential therapies appear promising, not all are at the same stage of development. Some neuroprotective drugs, including certain antioxidants and antiexcitotoxic drugs, are already being tested in humans for other purposes. Recently discovered molecules, such as those that control axon guidance, will require a great deal of basic and applied research before they can be developed into useful drugs. With so many potential therapies for spinal cord injury, investigators must carry out efficient preclinical tests to ensure that the most effective therapies proceed as rapidly as possible to clinical trials and, ultimately, to proven safety and usefulness. New animal models and better ways to monitor the success of treatments are essential to this process.

Clinical Trials

Randomized, controlled human clinical trials are the "gold standard" for revealing the benefits and drawbacks of a therapy. However, such trials are usually very expensive, and they are unlikely to yield useful results without adequate preclinical study. Clinical trials that do not yield clear answers are an enormous waste of resources. Physicians conducting clinical trials also must ensure that they do no harm to the patients in their study. The Belmont report of 1978, which guides human medical research ethics in the United States, reaffirmed that the rights of individuals participating in clinical trials must take precedence over the potential benefit to society as a whole. This restricts randomized trials to those therapies that have shown potential usefulness in systematic preclinical studies. Only with good preclinical data can researchers predict which treatment regimens might be useful and whether new therapies can be combined with standard therapy.

A clinical trial involves hundreds of components, all of which are important to its success. Seven components essential to a good trial include the rationale, or reasons the trial should be carried out; the design, which should compare different therapies (or therapy and placebo); the inclusion and exclusion criteria determining which patients should enter the trial; the use of randomization or bias control measures; the number of patients to be tested in order to produce clear results; carefully defined outcome events (that is, measures of how well patients recover); and the analysis of the data. For a clinical trial to be justified, physicians should ideally be in a state of "equipoise" in which they are not sure whether a treatment works or not. If they are certain a treatment works, it is unethical to withhold it from patients. Yet, without a reasonable expectation that patients will benefit, it is difficult to justify the risks.

There are three phases of systematic clinical testing in the United States. Phase I trials determine the criteria for safe and effective use of the therapy. These trials usually involve small numbers of patients and test the therapy in a range of doses. It is important to make this phase as extensive as necessary to eliminate unknown factors that can confound the results of later, more expensive phase II and III trials. Phase II trials establish whether the therapy, at safe and optimal doses, works for the disease. These trials should also help define factors such as which patients might benefit from the therapy. Finally, Phase III trials compare the new therapies to other therapies and/or to placebo. These trials are usually very large, as they must involve enough patients to reasonably show the drug's benefits and potential adverse reactions. A company must obtain phase III data before applying for FDA approval of a new drug.

The NASCIS trial that established the benefits of methylprednisolone is a model of an efficient phase III clinical trial for spinal cord therapy. This efficiency resulted from the trial's design, which used one placebo control group compared to two therapies: methylprednisolone and naloxone. This design made optimal use of resources, with a minimal number of patients given placebo. The NASCIS II trial also revealed that most patients improve somewhat, regardless of whether or not they receive methylprednisolone -- knowledge that is important for designing future clinical studies. Because methylprednisolone reduces disability, clinical trials can no longer use placebo controls because it would be unethical to withhold the drug from patients. Instead, new therapies must be compared to methylprednisolone, the best standard therapy.

A special problem in testing therapies for spinal cord injury is that most studies thus far have found combination therapies to be the most effective strategies. The need to test several therapies together complicates and can confound traditional clinical trial strategies. Investigators must find effective ways to deal with this problem to test many of the promising therapies for spinal cord injury.

Researchers have identified a wide variety of potential therapies for spinal cord injury. To efficiently evaluate these therapies, however, investigators need to carry out well-designed, preclinical and clinical studies. Key elements include cooperation between multiple independent research centers, strategic trial design, and well-defined criteria for selecting potential therapies to be tested. The success of the methylprednisolone trial and advances from the basic science realm have stimulated the pace of research on treating spinal cord injury. With properly designed trials, potential therapies can be efficiently tested so they can help people with spinal cord injuries as soon as possible.

Spinal cord injury research has now come of age. Because of general progress in neuroscience, as well as specific advances in spinal cord injury research, researchers can test new ideas about how changes in molecules, cells, and their complex interactions in the living body determine the outcome of spinal cord injury. Scientists are learning, for example, how processes such as oxidative damage, excitotoxicity, and apoptosis contribute to spinal cord injury and how this damage might be minimized. Inspired by demonstrations that spinal cord nerve cells can regrow, researchers are learning to manipulate trophic factors, intrinsic growth programs, and growth inhibitors to encourage regeneration.

One of the most exciting aspects of the workshop was the potential for applying findings from other fields, such as development, immunology, and stroke research, to spinal cord injury. There is increasing recognition that similar processes contribute to a diverse range of neurological disorders, including spinal cord injury, stroke, brain trauma, and neurodegenerative diseases. New insights about how the nervous system develops are also suggesting ways to encourage regeneration. Researchers may debate how directly these insights will apply to the adult spinal cord, but they agree that testing these hypotheses in animal models of spinal cord injury ultimately will lead to better treatments.

Overcoming spinal cord injuries will require general progress in many fields of neuroscience as well as specific studies in animal models of spinal cord injury and in patients themselves. Key areas for research include:

- Secondary damage and intrinsic repair processes, including oxidative damage, excitotoxicity, calcium-mediated damage, proteases, apoptosis, immune responses, stem cells, and plasticity and reorganization.
- Development and regeneration, including trophic factors, axonal pathfinding, growth inhibitors, and synapse formation.
- Applied studies in animal models of spinal cord injury, including tests of trophic factors and grafting and transplantation strategies.
- Clinical research in human patients, including studies to describe anatomical and functional changes that follow spinal cord injury, to refine existing supportive and rehabilitation therapies such as neural prostheses, and to test new therapies that emerge from basic and applied research.

Researchers are wary of giving people false hopes that a magic bullet for curing spinal cord injury is just around the corner. However, with accelerating progress in scientific research, there is renewed vitality and growing optimism that, with continued effort, the problems of spinal cord injury will be overcome.

Conclusion

Therapies for spinal cord injury have improved substantially in the last few years. Drugs for treatment of acute injury, neural prostheses, and advanced rehabilitation strategies are improving the survival and quality of life for many patients. However, there are still many opportunities for improvement. These include finding ways to build on CNS reorganization and comparing the usefulness of different rehabilitation strategies. Investigators must also develop improved animal models for spinal cord injury to allow testing of new or improved therapies.

Chapter 8

Newer Inventions

Introduction

For the first time, scientists have regenerated spinal cord nerves by removing a 'biological brake' on their growth -- a breakthrough that raises hope for thousands of patients left paralysed by back and neck injuries. Researchers at the Reeve-Irvine Research Centre in the US, focused on a protein that turns off the growth of nerve fibres in adults, using mice as test subjects. By genetically deleting the enzyme, they were able to switch the ability of the nerves to regenerate back on. The scientists are now investigating whether the technique can restore movement to mice crippled by spinal cord injuries, the Daily Mail reported.

"Paralysis and loss of function from spinal cord injury has been considered untreatable, but our discovery points the way towards a potential therapy to induce regeneration of nerve connections following spinal cord injury in people." Professor Steward is director of the Reeve-Irvine Research Centre, named after Christopher Reeve, the former 'Superman' star, who was paralysed from the neck down in a riding accident. It is dedicated to investigating treatments for spinal injury. According to scientists, an injury the size of a grape can lead to complete loss of function beneath the breakage point. Severed nerves, which control the voluntary movement, in the neck may cause paralysis of the arms and legs, and an inability to control the bladder and bowel. "All these functions could be restored if we could find a way to regenerate the connections that were damaged," said Professor Steward. The findings were reported in the journal Nature Neuroscience.

Twenty-year-old Melissa Holley loves swimming at the local pool near her home in Ridgway, Colo. She works out a few times a week. But she can no longer play soccer (she was a star player in high school), or dance. On June 25, 2000, driving from one of her waitress jobs to the other, she crashed while going around a curve. Police say she may have been speeding, and she wasn't wearing a seat belt. One of her vertebrae was crushed, and she was paralyzed from her mid-trunk down. "You, you don't believe it at first. You are just like, you know, no. I can get past this; it is just temporary, it's OK," says Holley.

Doctors have offered her parents, Gwen and Roy, essentially no hope that she ever would walk again. But her father would not accept it. Roy

Holley teaches leadership skills; within hours, he put his own to work, scanning the globe to prove the doctors wrong. He found information about a new treatment designed to repair nerve damage in patients with recent spinal cord injuries. But there was a catch. The treatment did have a great success rate, but so far only in the lab, and only in rats. There was another catch. While the FDA has approved a clinical trial of this treatment in the U.S., the only doctors actually using it were 7,000 miles away in Israel. Researchers there, at a company called Proneuron, had been looking for a suitable human patient for months. They couldn't believe it when Roy Holley simply called them out of the blue.

The Holleys borrowed $90,000 to get her to Israel within the treatment's two-week window.

The key to the research is macrophages, special immune cells that promote healing. But they are not found in great numbers in the spinal cord. The Israelis' revolutionary idea is to isolate them in another part of the patient's body, and then inject them into the damaged spinal cord. Doctors had never before considered this method, fearing it might aggravate the injury. How much she will improve, we don't know. We don't know. We don't know what to expect because she is the first one," says Dr. Valentine Fulga, who is leading the research

How much she will
improve, we don't know. We don't know. We don't know what to expect because she is the first one," says Dr. Valentine Fulga, who is leading the research.For 70 per cent of the rats, the cells helped the spinal nerves regenerate. Two weeks after the procedure, Melissa began to feel sensation in her legs. When she returned to Colorado, her progress continued. "Slowly but surely it... it, you

know, spread to my ,you know, abdomen and stomach and my lower back," she says.

Her ability to move has also returned, although more slowly. Now, less than a year after her accident, Melissa can lift her once-paralyzed legs. Her Israeli surgeon, Nachshon Knoller, believes that she will walk again. Doctors say that if this new procedure does work for Melissa, it might work for other patients with recent spinal cord injuries. "I'll never be satisfied until I am the way I was," says Melissa

Cell and Gene Therapies: Strategies for Spinal Cord Injury

"The neural circuitry in the CNS (central nervous system) is basically a simple system: you need to get information up to the brain, and you need to send information down to the spinal cord," said Howard Nornes, PhD, professor in the Department of Anatomy and Neurobiology at Colorado State University and consultant for the new Spinal Cord Society (SCS) Research Center in Fort Collins, Colorado. Dr. Nornes' talk, "Cell and Gene Therapies: Strategies for SCI," was sponsored by the SCS.

"Each segment of the spinal cord has the same basic neuronal circuitry," he continued. "The primary sensory neurons in the dorsal root ganglia transmit information from the body into the segment; the motor neurons located in the ventral horn of the segment transmit information from the spinal cord to muscles; the ascending projection neurons transmit information from the segment to the brain; finally, the descending projection neurons located in the brain transmit information from the brain to each particular spinal segment."

The nerve cells involved in processing information are called neurons. Each neuron has a nerve cell body, dendrites that receive inputs (information), and a long fiber called an axon that carries signals from the cell body. When a segment of the spinal cord is injured, some of the axons passing through that segment are damaged. But even if the axon is damaged, the cell body may survive. "I think this is an important issue," Nornes said. "It turns out that in experimental animals, the cell bodies of long tract neurons to the spinal cord survive. This is good news as it is the cell bodies that are required for activating regeneration." Replacing damaged cells and the connections between cells in the nervous system is the focus of much nerve regeneration research today. Nornes has approached this problem first by trying to understand what happens when cells are transplanted into the adult nervous system.

In one experiment, Nornes' team made a cavity in a rat spinal cord, implanted embryonic neurons into the cavity, and found they survived and grew fibers into the host. Next he wanted to know–Can these implanted neurons do anything meaningful? Can they actually restore a function? Nornes addressed these questions in an experiment using the hind limb reflex system of the rat. In this system, stimulating a specific area in the brainstem will cause the hind leg to flex, which can be measured with a force transducer attached to the foot. If the area in the brainstem is damaged, the reflex function is lost. In his rat experiments, Nornes removed the cells responsible for this reflex, replaced them with embryonic cells, and found that the reflex came back. "This is a demonstration which shows that when you put a cell in the adult nervous system, it survives, it grows fibers, and in this case it restored a specific function," he said.

Another experiment involved making a bridge across the damaged area of the spinal cord. Nornes lesioned the rat spinal cord, implanted embryonic spinal cord tissue, allowed it to heal, and found that the implant formed tissue continuity with the host tissue. "This shows that implanted cells in the spinal cord grow and fill up the space," Nornes said. However, a slide magnifying the transplant area showed that few fibers grow into the transplant from the host. "This again illustrates that few adult neurons are able to regenerate," he said.

Many researchers have been working on this problem. "People have transplanted peripheral nerve cells and embryonic cells. They've used synthetic matrixes. They've added growth factors and antibodies. And in spite of doing all these kinds of things, there is minimal growth of host axons into the transplants," Nornes said. "This is a fundamental issue that we have to deal with to accomplish meaningful regeneration and recovery of function in the injured spinal cord." One approach has been to try to understand and replicate the process by which growth occurs in the nervous system during embryonic development.

"During the development of the nervous system, growth genes are upregulated and drive the growth of the neurons," Nornes said. Once the nervous system is wired up (all the connections are established), this growth program is shut down.

"Our challenge is to identify the key genes that are involved in activating growth, understand how to regulate them, and then regulate them to activate growth," Nornes said. "The tools of molecular biology are able to accomplish this. It is possible to isolate a particular gene, characterize how to regulate that gene (turn it off or on), and finally, apply appropriate treatments to modify gene expression." Nornes gave an example of how his research team accomplished this in an experimental SCI model in rats. He and his research team modified the expression of a gene involved in making neurons receptive to a growth factor. After applying the gene treatment to cells in experimentally injured adult rat spinal cords, he was able to measure an improvement in locomotion and strength. "It was a slight improvement," said Nornes. Nonetheless, "these experiments show that it is possible to make gene-targeted treatments in spinal cord injuries."

While the results are very exciting and promising, Nornes insists that a great deal more work needs to be done. "The good news is that as we learn more about cells and how they can be made responsive to growth factors, we will be able to isolate and regulate and treat the appropriate neurons and activate growth." The SCS Research Center is staffed and equipped to investigate the problems of chronic SCI at the cellular and molecular level. "What is different at this point in history is that we have the tools to work with this problem at the molecular level," said Nornes. "I think the progress that will be made in the next five years will be very significant in contrast to the last 30 years. It's an extremely exciting time."

Chapter 9

Rehabilitation

Spinal Cord Injury Implications and Occupational Therapy

The signs and symptoms of spinal cord injury (SCI) significantly impact everyday activities. Occupational therapy plays an important role in the rehabilitation and management of SCI at all levels. An important therapeutic goal is to assist the client to restore function, enabling clients' to participate in the activities and tasks that are important to them. The ability to participate in meaningful, everyday activities is essential to an individual's health and well-being. Occupational therapists (OTs) focus on three life areas, which include self-care, productivity, and leisure. Self-care tasks include basic needs such as **bathing, hygiene, feeding, and dressing. Productivity** includes activities such as paid work, volunteering, caregiving, or parenting. Leisure includes fun and enjoyable activities activities typically done during spare time. Performing daily activities can be difficult for an individual with a spinal cord injury. However, through the rehabilitation process individuals with SCI can live independently in the community with or without full-time attendant care, depending on the level of their injury. [13]

Occupational therapist's work collaboratively with their clients to identify challenges in the performance of daily tasks and activities related to self-care, productivity and leisure. [14] Informal and formal assessments help OTs gain information that helps them to understand their clients' challenges.

How Occupational Therapy Can Help Address Occupational Performance Issues

When an individual receives occupational therapy, they are referred to as a client. The role of occupational therapy in SCI rehabilitation is to assist clients in regaining abilities and roles that are important and meaningful. [15] After identifying areas that the client feels challenged with, the OT and client work together to prioritize and set goals. Together, they create plans that address the performance issues in order to encourage participation in everyday activities. An important feature of occupational therapy is the use of 'therapeutic activities' to achieve this goal. Finally, reassessment is done to measure the outcome of the effectiveness of the therapy plans.

Pallastrini et al [15] emphasize the importance of early occupational therapy, started immediately after the client is stable. During these early stages, OTs evaluate what the client is able to do and what the client is having difficulty with. Occupational therapists then work one-on-one with the client on skills required for daily living. The client is shown new ways of doing things and may be given assistive devices or equipment. Occupational therapists also help their clients develop coping skills, and implement exercises and routines that strengthen muscles. [15]

Occupational therapists use the information gained from formal and informal assessments to guide their intervention plans. When considering the role of OT in SCI, it is helpful to think about what interventions are commonplace during different phases of recovery, namely acute, acute rehabilitation and community phases. During the rehabilitation process, assessments are re-administered to evaluate progress and the effectiveness of therapy interventions. When considering assessments and interventions, consideration must also be given to age, gender, and a multitude of client-specific factors.

Phase 1: Acute Recovery

During acute recovery, the focus is on support and prevention. The OT helps the client gain a sense of control over a situation in which the client likely feels little independence. [13] The OT may make splints to prevent deformities in the hands. Additionally, daily arm and hand exercises are performed to maintain normal function. Fitting and selecting the most appropriate temporary wheelchair to enable mobility is important in this stage. Finally, teaching the client and care providers appropriate positioning in bed and in the wheelchair is critical for the prevention of pressure sores. [13] Education regarding pressure sore prevention continues into the rehabilitation phase. See self-care skills.

Phase 2: Acute Rehabilitation

During acute rehabilitation, OT interventions focus on support, education for the client and family/caregivers, meaningful activities, choosing equipment and restoring the client's self esteem and confidence. [13] It is particularly important to consider the client's discharge environment (i.e. home, community and social setting) in order to prepare for community living. With the client, the OT creates an individual program to meet the client's needs. The following are key areas of intervention common to numerous rehabilitation settings [16] :

Assessment and treatment of the upper limbs.

Early in the rehabilitation phase, the OT evaluates the client's strength and sensation in the upper extremity (UE); lower extremity (LE) evaluation falls under the responsibility of the physical therapist. The OT makes use of therapeutic activities to both strengthen muscles and improve hand function. Custom-made splints are commonly used to help position the hands in a functional position and assist in preventing deformity. [16] Individuals who retain wrist function are taught to use tenodesis grasp (extending the wrist to bring the thumb and index finger together and flexing the wrist to separate the thumb and index finger) for picking up and releasing light objects. [13] Using meaningful activities to build strength, endurance, and coordination helps to differentiate the work of occupational therapists from physical therapists.

Self care retraining.

Obtaining competency in self-care tasks contributes significantly to an individual's sense of self confidence and independence. The focus is on feeding, grooming, bathing, dressing and bowel/bladder management. [13] Assistive devices and specialized equipment are prescribed by the OT to help the client achieve greater competency and independence in their activities of daily living. Depending on the level and severity of the injury, independence in feeding, grooming, UE dressing and bathing may be achieved with the assistance of adaptive equipment for dressing and bathing the LE.

[17] Examples of commonly prescribed equipment include: dressing and bathing aids for the LE, a padded transfer tub bench, shower-commode chair, or hand-held shower. Adaptive devices may also be required to assist with bowel and bladder management. A key role for the OT is to educate both the client and the client's caregiver(s) in the proper care and use of the adaptive aids/equipment. Practice sessions under the supervision and guidance of the OT are provided until the client feels competent using the adaptive aids and techniques.

Pressure sores are secondary complications of SCI. Educating clients about the risks that lead to pressure sores and strategies for prevention is important to health and well-being.[16] For example, an important part of the prevention strategy includes teaching clients about the importance of maintaining a good position in bed and in any seating aids (e.g. wheelchair). In addition, the OT teaches the client about the importance of shifting their weight regularly in both lying and seated positions. Clients who lack strength in their upper extremity can achieve a weight shift by tilting their chair in space. Tilting the wheelchair takes pressure off the buttocks area, which is one area at high-risk for pressure sore development. In addition to education, the therapist assesses the client for the best pressure relieving surfaces (i.e. cushion and mattress) to aid in pressure sore prevention.

Transfer skills.

Transfers are a key area of education and skill development. [16] Examples of different transfers include: moving from bed to wheelchair, from wheelchair to toilet or tub, and from wheelchair to driver's seat. Strength in the upper extremities makes it possible to transfer independently from one surface to another either with the aid of a sliding transfer board or by utilizing grab bars. Frequent practice under the guidance of the OT assists clients with the necessary skill development.

Bed mobility.

Occupational therapists teach their clients bed mobility skills required for many daily tasks, such as getting dressed, moving out of bed, and correct positioning in bed for skin protection and comfort. [16]

Mobility skills.

Not being able to move around without help is the largest restriction to participating in activities of daily living. The wheelchair that a person uses can significantly affect their quality of participation. A key area for the OT is to assist clients with the selection of the most suitable mobility aid in accordance with their needs, finances, abilities, preferences and available technology. [18] A proper fitting wheelchair is critical for good posture and comfort. Creating an ideal match between the client's needs and the equipment available is challenging. The client's level of funding and the high cost of equipment adds further complexity. [18]

The level and severity of a clients SCI determines the most suitable mobility aid. For example, some clients require a power wheelchair both indoors and outdoors while others can manage on both terrains using a manual wheelchair. If a client requires assistance with uneven outdoor surfaces, the OT may prescribe both a power and manual wheelchair to allow for flexibility according to their needs. This involves fitting clients for both wheelchairs and selecting the best pressure relieving surfaces/cushions and backrests. In addition, power and manual wheelchair training assists clients in developing skills both indoors and outdoors.

Home assessment and modifications.

Discussing the client's housing situation is an important part of rehabilitation planning. Where possible, the OT will make a home visit to assess the need for changes and adaptations to the home. Examples of common adaptations include: adding ramps or lifts to get into the home, widening doorways, adapting the bathroom and kitchen for wheelchair accessibility, placing electrical switches at wheelchair level, and choosing wheelchair-friendly flooring. Involving the client and family in determining solutions and making decisions is very important. Assessing the need for specialized equipment (i.e. hospital bed or pressure relieving mattress) also takes place during rehabilitation. The client will be encouraged to try different pieces of equipment in relation to self-care, communication, and other activities of daily living. With guidance from the OT, the client will decide on the most appropriate items of equipment to suit their needs.[21]

Domestic retraining.

During rehabilitation, opportunities are provided for clients to practice a variety of domestic skills. For example, clients can practice cooking in a wheelchair-accessible kitchen. They can trial different pieces of equipment that can enhance independence in this area. A variety of adaptive aids for the kitchen address limitations in grip strength. [15] Occupational therapists teach adaptive strategies for carrying out domestic chores (i.e. childcare, cleaning, laundry) that are adjusted to suit the client's needs and abilities. It may be necessary to hire a community home care support worker to assist with domestic chores. The amount of additional outside support depends on the level and severity of the client's SCI and can vary from 24 hours per day to just a few hours per day. [13]

Assistance with return to driving/transportation.

Clients who are able to transfer independently from their wheelchair to the driver's seat using a sliding transfer board, are candidates for returning to driving. Complete independence with driving also requires the ability to load and unload one's wheelchair from the vehicle. [13] Clients capable of driving are referred by the OT to the 'Return to driving program' within the Driver Assessment and Rehabilitation Unit at the hospital. The goal of the program is to provide education and retraining to help clients return to driving. Assistance with selecting an appropriate modified vehicle that will meet the client's needs and budget are part of the program. For clients who do not wish to return to driving, alternate transportation options are also addressed (i.e. accessible parking, taxi subsidy vouchers, modified vehicle for passenger transit and public transportation).

Community living skills.

Clients may be involved in a support group, which addresses skills that prepare clients for returning home and to the community. As previously mentioned, driving and wheelchair mobility skills are important for accessing the community. Community outings are commonly organized to help transition the client into the community. [16] (See community reintegration for more details.)

Leisure and recreation skills.

Part of rehabilitation involves investigating options for returning to previous leisure/recreation interests as well as developing new pursuits. In addition, the OT can assist the client in finding ways to cope with physical and social issues that may get in the way of leisure participation. [17]

Work/study skills.

Addressing the client's career and educational goals is very important. If appropriate, a work site/school visit may be arranged to assess for accessibility. Otherwise, a referral to a community based work/school assessment service may be indicated. [17]

Sexual Health.

Exploring concerns related to sexual health and function should form an integral part of each client's treatment plan. The OT can assist their client by providing information and identifying alternate resources and adaptive devices as needed. [17]

Phase 3: Community reintegration

Following rehabilitation, the client begins the process of community reintegration. Community participation is an important aspect in maintaining quality of life. [19] During community reintegration, the focus of occupational therapy is on restoring client roles at home and in the community, and promoting social participation and life satisfaction. [19] Ongoing education of the client, family and caregivers continues throughout this stage. Referrals can be made to an outpatient clinic or community therapist to continue with treatment and progress made during rehabilitation.

Outpatient programs teach clients how to use new movement and they offer training for activities of daily living as clients continue to gain strength during the first year after injury. In addition, the OT and client work on goals and skills that encourage the client towards community integration (i.e. driving, vocational evaluation and training, participation in leisure interests). Additionally, the therapist identifies transitional services such as support groups and transitional living centres if required.

Occupational therapists are also involved with advocacy on behalf of their clients. Advocacy can take many forms and apply in areas that impact the client's ability to fully participate within their community. This includes helping to address barriers to employment, and leisure at a policy level. Examples of large barriers involving physical structures are playground designs, city planning, and accessible buildings. An OT can address decision makers, argue in favour of their client's needs and bring important information and perspectives to others who may be causing a barrier for the client. Occupational therapists can promote awareness, and lobby on behalf of their clients. Finally, OTs address issues such as social stigma by advocating on their client's behalf. Stigma can be addressed: (a) by challenging others to think differently, (b) by making others aware of marginalization, and (c) by helping others understand the loss of privileges that can occur at both the societal and policy level. [20]

- Brown-Sequard Syndrome
- Syringomyelia
- Paraplegia
- Quadriplegia/Tetraplegia

External links

- Miami Project to Cure Paralysis Noted for experimental cooling protocol used on Kevin Everett
- United Spinal Association A membership organization dedicated to improving the quality of life of individuals with spinal cord injuries and related disorders.

- Syringomyelia Foundation A Non-Profit Charity whose goal is to improve the quality of life of those who suffer from Syringomyelia (also known as Morvan's Disease) and other spinal cord injuries and conditions by providing various types of assistance as needed on a case-by-case basis through case management
- Rehabilitation Research and Training Center (RRTC) on Spinal Cord Injury: Promoting Health and Preventing Complications through Exercise
- SCI Images - Images of Spinal Cord Injury
- sci.rutgers.edu - Spinal Cord Injury Levels and Classification

- The Spinal Cord Injury Project, W.M. Keck Center for Collaborative Neuroscience at Rutgers University
- EMSCI Network European Multicenter Study about Spinal Cord Injury
- Brigham and Women's Hospital Translational Pain Research Clinical trials for pain following SCI
- Pediatric and Adolescent Spinal Cord Injury
- Rehabilitation Engineering Research Center on Wheeled Mobility
- International Institute for Research in Paraplegia Research funding foundation, based in Zurich
- Spinal Cord Injuries Emergency Medicine for Spinal Cord Injuries

- Trefethen, Tre. User's Manual for the Paralyzed Penis: Love after spinal cord injury American Sexuality Magazine. Accessed 3-22-07.
- About Spinal Cord Injury Spinal Cord Injury FAQ for those with SCI, and their families, by Canadian Paraplegic Association - Ontario.
- ICF based Case studies in Spinal Cord Injury Rehabilitation
- CareCure Community Social and informational site for individuals with spinal cord injuries.
- Spinal Cord Injury Health Information Information and support for people affected

  With spinal cord injuries

References

1. Spinal Cord Medicine: Principles and Practice (2002) Lin VWH, Cardenas DD, Cutter NC, Frost FS, Hammond MC. Demos Medical Publishing
2. Spinal Cord Medicine (2001) Kirshblum S, Campagnolo D, Delisa J. Lippincott Williams & Wilkins
3. http://www.fscip.org/facts.htm
4. Qiu J (July 2009). "China Spinal Cord Injury Network: changes from within". *Lancet Neurol* **8** (7): 606–7. doi:10.1016/S1474-4422(09)70162-0. PMID 19539234.
5. Klebin, Phil Sexual Function of Men with Spinal Cord Injury May 2007
6. "UpToDate Inc.". http://www.uptodate.com/online/conte

nt/topic.do?topicKey=medneuro/10703&selectedTitle=3~150&source=search_result.

7. "BestBets: Steroids in acute spinal cord injury". http://www.bestbets.org/bets/bet.php?id=105.

8. Abraham S (March 2008). "Autologous Stem Cell Injections for Spinal Cord Injury - A multicentric Study with 6 month follow up of 108 patients". *7th Annual Meeting of Japanese Society of Regenerative Medicine, Nagoya, Japan.*

9. R Ravikumar, S Narayanan and S Abraham (Nov 2007). "Autologous stem cells for spinal cord injury". *Regenerative Medicine* **2** (6): 53-61.

10. Abraham S (June 2007). "Autologous Bone Marrow Mononuclear Cells for spinal cord injury- A case report". *Cytotherapy* **9** (1).

11. Dobkin, BH.; Curt, A.; Guest, J. "Cellular transplants in China: observational study from the largest human experiment in chronic spinal cord injury." Neurorehabilitation and Neural Repair, v. 20 issue 1, 2006, p. 5-13.

12. Krupa T, Fossey E, Anthony WA, Brown C. Doing daily life: how occupational therapy can inform psychiatric rehabilitation practice. Psychiatr Rehabil J.2009; 32(3), 155-161.

13. Radomski MV, Trombly Latham CA. Occupational therapy for physical dysfunction: 6th ed. Baltimore, MD: Lippincott Williams & Wilkins; 2008.

14. Canadian Association of Occupational Therapists. Enabling occupation: an occupational therapy perspective (Rev. ed.). Ottawa, (ON): CAOT Publications ACE; 2002.

15. Pillastrini P, Mugnai R, Bonfiglioli R, Curti S, Mattioli S, Maioli MG, et al. Evaluation of an occupational therapy program for patients with spinal cord injury. Spinal Cord 2008;46:78-81.

16. Ozelie R, Sipple S, Foy T, Cantoni K, Kellogg K, Lookingbill J, et al. Classification of SCI

rehabilitation treatments #8: SCI Rehab Project Series: The Occupational Therapy Taxonomy. J Spinal Cord Med 2009;32:283–297.

17. Atchison BJ, Dirette, D.K. Conditions in Occupational Therapy. Effect on Occupational Performance. 3rd ed. Baltimore, MD: Lippincott Williams & Wilkins; 2007.

18. Di Marco A, Russell M, Masters M. Standards for wheelchair prescription. Aust Occup Ther J 2003;50:30-39.

19. Cohen ME, Schemm RL. Client-centered occupational therapy for individuals with Spinal Cord Injury. Occup Ther in Health Care 2007;21(3):1-15.

20. Townsend EA, Polatajko H. Enabling occupation II: Advancing an occupational therapy vision for health, well-being, & justice through occupation. Ottawa, Ontario: CAOT Publications; 2007.
21. http://wikipedia.unicefuganda.org/latest/A/Spinal cord injury

Chapter: 10

Conclusion

Research in spinal cord regeneration is catching attention of clinicians and basic scientists. It would almost revolutionise the life and disease outcome of these unfortunate patients if we can work out a cost effective and practical treatment regimen for these victims who are unfortunately in the prime of their productive years. It was gratifying to learn that nerves in peripheral nervous system (PNS), which are outside the brain or spinal cord, did regrow. It is exciting to learn that the prospects of regrowth of spinal cord improve when these PNS cells are implanted in damaged spinal cord. Spinal cord injury is a global epidemic. A lot of research is going on in this field. Axonal regeneration, electric stimulation, Netrins, stem cells etc are few exciting fields in the area of research. It is ongoing research whereby the ability to grow human motor neurons in the laboratory will provide new insights into disease processes and could be used as alternative to animal models for finding therapeutic targets and testing drug.

Researchers have identified a wide variety of potential therapies for spinal cord injury. To efficiently evaluate these therapies, however, investigators need to carry out well-designed preclinical and clinical trials that will reveal the benefits and drawbacks of each strategy.

While all of these potential therapies appear promising, not all are at the same stage of development. Some neuroprotective drugs, including certain antioxidants and antiexcitotoxic drugs, are already being tested in humans for other purposes. Recently discovered molecules, such as those that control axon guidance, will require a great deal of basic and applied research before they can be developed into useful drugs. With so many potential therapies for spinal cord injury, investigators must carry out efficient preclinical tests to ensure that the most effective therapies proceed as rapidly as possible to clinical trials and, ultimately, to proven safety and usefulness. New animal models and better ways to monitor the success of treatments are essential to this process.

A lot has been done. A lot needs to be done. It is the principal responsibility of planners, politicians, sociologists, scientists, researchers to contribute all their might to work on strategies to reduce mortality, contain morbidity and eventually make these unfortunate victms live the life of ordinary denizens. In his humanity can raise its head again!!!!!

About The Authors

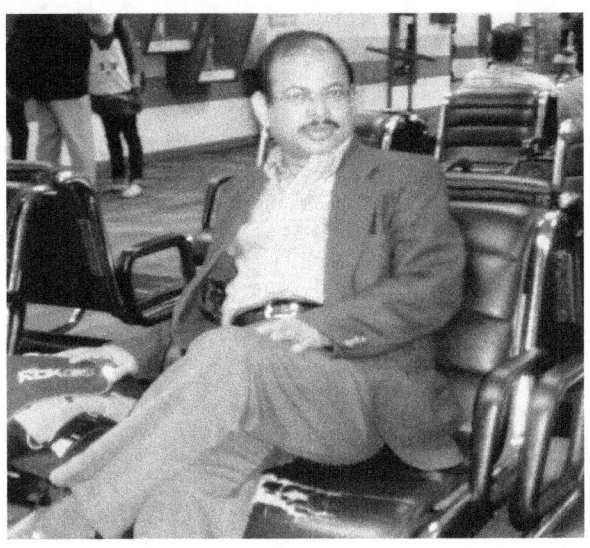

Dr Gourishankar Patnaik

Prof (Dr) Gourishankar Patnaik was born on the 28th August 1960 at Cuttack, Orissa. He had his schooling in the central Indian town of Nagpur. Maintaining a brilliant academic career and being in the top 10 students in the state in the higher secondary certificate examination he entered in the prestigious Government Medical College, Nagpur in 1977. He graduated in 1981-82 being the best graduate of the Nagpur University with seven gold medals which was a record haul. He had distinction in surgery, obstetrics and Gynecology and Preventive and Social Medicine. He finished his Masters in Orthopedics (M.S.) from Nagpur University in 1986.

He has subsequently worked in Govt. medical College Nagpur, Annamalai University, Ministry of Health, and Oman. He was Formerly Professor of Orthopedic surgery at Institute of Medical sciences, Bhubaneshwar and until recently was the Professor and Head of the prestigious Manipal University in Malaysia at their international Medical College in Melaka, Malaysia. Presently he is the Professor and Head Dept Of Trauma, Orthopedics and Rehabilitation Narayan Medical College Hospital Jamuhar, Bihar.

Dr Patnaik holds AO trauma fellowship from the University of Alabama, Birmingham, USA. He had many training stints in Europe, Singapore, and Middle East. He holds a postgraduate degree in Public administration, Sociology and Economics. Widely travelled, his research interests include E learning, Distance learning, Spinal injuries, Diabetes and arthritis.

He is on the board of many social organizations. He has authored many books and is a prolific orator and teacher.

About the Author

Dr kumar Anshuman

Dr Kumar Anshuman is a young and dynamic orthopaedic surgeon with interest in trauma, spinal injuries and arthroscopy.He has his orthopeic training at Sir Gangaram Hospital where he finished his DNB orthopaedics with Distinction.He is a senior Assistant Professor in orthopaedic surgery atthe Narayan Medical College and hospital, Sasaram, Bihar India. He is the son of eminent orthopedic surgeon Dr Darbari Singh.

Books Authored By Prof Gourishankar Patnaik

1. The Aging Knee
2. Osteoporosis : The Silent Killer
3. Understanding Stress: Effective Management Techniques
4. E learning: Scopes and Limitations
5. Musculoskeletal Manifestations in Diabetes Mellitus
6. Overuse Injuries in Orthopedic Practice
7. Musculoskeletal Medicine for undergraduate
8. Orthopedics for undergraduate
9. Understanding anger: Effective management Techniques
10. Cissus Quadrangularis: a wonder herb
11. Understanding Death : Theological Perspectives
12. Understanding Diabetic Foot
13. Art Of Dying :Can Death be a Celebration
14. **Understanding Women**

Notes....

www.ingramcontent.com/pod-product-compliance
Lightning Source LLC
Chambersburg PA
CBHW051643170526
45167CB00001B/309